AMERICAN ACADEMY OF PEDIATRICS

GUIDE TO YOUR CHILD'S ALLERGIES AND ASTHMA

D1411601

CHILDCARE BOOKS FROM THE AMERICAN ACADEMY OF PEDIATRICS

AMERICAN ACADEMY OF PEDIATRICS

GUIDE TO YOUR CHILD'S ALLERGIES AND ASTHMA

Breathing Easy and Bringing Up Healthy, Active Children

EDITOR-IN-CHIEF

Michael J. Welch, M.D., FAAP
Allergy & Asthma Medical Group & Research Center
San Diego, California

Villard
New York

Libary of Congress Cataloging-in-Publication Data
American Academy of Pediatrics guide to your child's asthma and allergies: breathing easy and bringing up healthy, active children / Michael J. Welch, editor-in-chief
      p. cm.
Includes index.
ISBN: 0-679-76982-X
1. Asthma in children—Popular works. 2. Allergy in children—Popular works. I. Title: Guide to your child's asthma and allergies. II. Welch, Michael J. III. American Academy of Pediatrics.
RJ436.A8 A48 2000
618.92238—dc21

Random House Web site address: www.villard.com

Printed in the United States of America on acid-free paper

98765432

First Edition

Dedication

This book is dedicated to all the people who recognize that children are our greatest inspiration in the present and our greatest hope for the future.

From the Editor-in-Chief:

Dedicated to the many children out there who are:

The sneezers and wheezers
The sniffers and whiffers

The scratchers and rashers
The coughers and hackers

The itchers and twitchers
The snorers and blowers

Relief is in sight
In the pages just right

Hoping a look at this book
Was all that it took.

MJW

Reviewers/Contributors

Editor-in-Chief
Michael J. Welch, M.D., FAAP

AAP Board of Directors Reviewer
James E. Shira, M.D., FAAP

American Academy of Pediatrics

Executive Director
Joe M. Sanders, Jr., M.D., FAAP

Associate Executive Director
Roger F. Suchyta, M.D., FAAP

Director, Department of Education
Robert Perelman, M.D., FAAP

Director, Division of Public Education
Lisa R. Reisberg

Manager, Consumer Publishing
Division of Public Education
Brent L. Heathcott

Coordinator, Consumer Publishing
Division of Public Education
Veronica L. Noland

Reviewers/Contributors
A. Wesley Burks, M.D., FAAP
Louis Mendelson, M.D., FAAP
Thomas F. Plaut, M.D., FAAP
Hugh A. Sampson, M.D., FAAP
Diane Schuller, M.D., FAAP
Jay E. Selcow, M.D., FAAP
Laurie Smith, M.D., FAAP
Robert A. Wood, M.D., FAAP

Acknowledgments
Editorial production by DSH
Editorial, Inc., a division of
G.S. Sharpe Communications, Inc.

Editorial Director
Genell J. Subak-Sharpe, M.S.

Writers
Rosemary Perkins
Genell J. Subak-Sharpe, M.S.

Copy Editor
Karen Richardson

Designers
Tanya Krawciw
Peter Lukic
Debra Rabinowitz

Illustrators
Peter Lukic
Briar Lee Mitchell

Desktop Publishing
Debra Rabinowitz

Guide to Your Child's Allergies and Asthma

PLEASE NOTE

The information contained in this book is intended to complement, not substitute for, the advice of your child's pediatrician. Before starting any treatment or program affecting your child's health and behavior, you should consult your own pediatrician, who can discuss your child's individual needs with you and counsel you about symptoms and treatments.

The information and advice in this book apply equally to children of both sexes. We have elected to alternate the use of "he" and "she" instead of using a single gender pronoun or the "he/she" construction. When a problem is more common in one gender than the other, it is indicated. Otherwise, you should assume that either gender can be equally affected, even though only one is referred to in the text.

FOREWORD

The American Academy of Pediatrics (AAP) welcomes you to the latest in its series of parenting books, *Guide to Your Child's Allergies and Asthma*.

Although allergies and asthma can develop at any age, they most commonly show up during childhood or early adulthood. These conditions are explored in detail in *Guide to Your Child's Allergies and Asthma*. This book will help parents identify and avoid allergen and asthma triggers; prevent asthma attacks in their children; evaluate traditional and alternative forms of treatment and therapy; and understand how to alleviate and prevent symptoms.

What separates this book from other reference books on allergies and asthma is that pediatricians who specialize in these disorders have extensively reviewed it. Under the direction of our editor-in-chief, the material in this book was developed with the assistance of numerous reviewers and contributors from the American Academy of Pediatrics and its committees and sections. Because medical information is constantly changing, every effort has been made to ensure that this book contains the most up-to-date findings. Readers may want to visit the AAP Web site at www.aap.org to keep current on this and other subjects.

It is the Academy's hope that this book will become an invaluable resource and reference guide to parents. We are confident that parents and caregivers will find the book extremely valuable. We encourage its use along with the advice and counsel of our readers' pediatricians, who will provide individual guidance and assistance related to the health of children.

The AAP is an organization of 55,000 primary care pediatricians, pediatric medical subspecialists, and pediatric surgical specialists dedicated to the health, safety, and well-being of infants, children, adolescents, and young adults. *Guide to Your Child's Allergies and Asthma* is part of the Academy's ongoing educational efforts to provide parents and caregivers with high-quality information on a broad spectrum of children's health issues.

Joe M. Sanders, Jr., M.D., FAAP
Executive Director

AMERICAN ACADEMY OF PEDIATRICS

GUIDE TO YOUR CHILD'S
ALLERGIES AND ASTHMA

Part I

The Basics

CHAPTER 1

Allergies and Asthma Explained

Every fall, 5-year-old Timmy develops a runny nose, itchy, puffy eyes, and attacks of sneezing. His mother shares the problem, which she dismisses as mild hay fever, and something her son has to learn to live with. Lately, however, Timmy has also suffered attacks of wheezing and shortness of breath when he visits his grandmother and plays with her cats. Timmy's pediatrician suspects allergic asthma, and wants him to undergo some tests.

At first, Maria Lopez thought her baby daughter had heat rash. But the dry, itchy patches didn't go away, and even though Maria put mittens on little Jenine's hands, she couldn't prevent the baby from rubbing and scratching the rashy areas until they were raw and infected.

Allergies and asthma often start in childhood and persist throughout life. Although neither can be cured, with understanding and proper care they can usually be kept under control.

When 6-year-old Tanisha Evans developed red, itchy eyes, her mother assumed she had caught pinkeye (infectious conjunctivitis) from a school friend. Her pediatrician prescribed antibiotic eyedrops, but 2 weeks later, Tanisha's eyes were as red and itchy as ever, leading her pediatrician to suspect allergic conjunctivitis rather than an infection.

At age 15, Joshua collapsed after being stung by a bee while on a Boy Scout camping trip. Fortunately, after a previous severe allergic reaction to bee venom, Joshua's allergy specialist had prescribed an epinephrine (adrenaline) autoinjector. Joshua followed the doctor's instructions and kept it with him at all times in case of such an emergency. Realizing he was having an attack of anaphylaxis, Joshua was able to get out the autoinjector and give himself a life-saving shot of epinephrine.

Then there's 7-year-old Jamie, who breaks out in itchy hives after eating peanuts. And 12-year-old Allison, who is left gasping for breath whenever she has to run a mile in her gym class.

— ❖ —

Although these brief case histories, culled from actual medical records, describe very different symptoms and situations, they have a common thread: All are related to allergies, which doctors sometimes call atopic diseases or hypersensitivity reactions. Indeed, allergies and asthma, which typically start in childhood, are by far the most common chronic diseases among children in the United States. Consider these statistics:

- Some 50 million Americans have allergies, or about 15 percent of the population.
- The most common type of allergy is hay fever (allergic rhinitis); the medical cost of treating it now exceeds $2 billion a year.
- More than 17 million Americans have asthma, and about one-fourth of these are under age 18. Asthma accounts for about 5,000 deaths a year.
- Seventy to 80 percent of children with asthma also have allergies, which are among the most common triggers for asthma.
- If one parent has allergies, there's a 25 percent chance that a child will also be allergic. The risk is more than doubled to 60 to 70 percent if both parents have allergies.

Many aspects of allergies and asthma still are not fully understood. But advances in the diagnosis and treatment of these disorders are helping millions of sufferers. These will be discussed in the following chapters. But first, here's a brief overview of these all-too-common chronic disorders.

WHAT ARE ALLERGIES?

Many people mistakenly use the word "allergy" to refer to almost any unpleasant or adverse reaction. We often hear someone say, "He's allergic to hard work," or "She's allergic to anything that's green." In reality, however, an allergic reaction usually is due to an overactive immune system. This system is made up of a number of organs throughout the body—principally the bone marrow, the thymus gland (which is located behind the breastbone in the upper chest), and a network of lymph nodes and lymph tissue scattered throughout the body, including the spleen, tonsils, and the adenoid, a gland at the top of the throat.

Normally, it's the immune system that protects the body against disease by searching out and destroying foreign invaders, such as viruses and bacteria. In an allergic reaction, the immune system overreacts and goes into action against a normally harmless substance, such as pollen or animal dander. These allergy-provoking substances are called allergens.

The bone marrow serves as a factory and storage house for white blood cells (leukocytes), as well as other types of blood cells. Some types of immature white blood cells, called stem cells, are carried to other parts of the immune system, where they develop into more specialized, disease-fighting cells. For example, T lymphocytes, or simply T-cells, complete their development in the thymus, an organ located behind the breastbone that is made up of lymphoid tissue. Mature T-cells attack invading micro-organisms directly.

B lymphocytes, or B-cells, develop in the lymph nodes and other lymphatic tissue. These cells produce antibodies—highly specialized proteins that are programmed to recognize a specific foreign invader and go into action to destroy it whenever it enters the body. These antibodies are useful and beneficial to the body.

In a person with allergies, the immune system also produces antibodies against allergens; these antibodies are not felt to be useful and actually lead to the various allergic problems that plague children and adults. Here is a simplified overview of what happens in a typical allergic response:

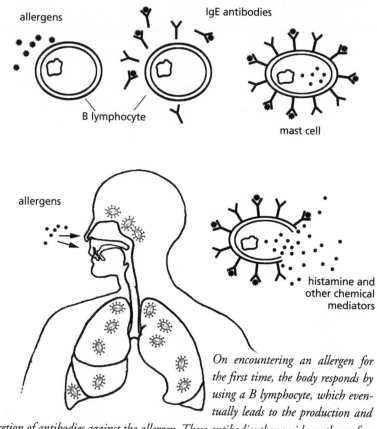

allergens

IgE antibodies

B lymphocyte

mast cell

allergens

histamine and other chemical mediators

On encountering an allergen for the first time, the body responds by using a B lymphocyte, which eventually leads to the production and secretion of antibodies against the allergen. These antibodies then reside on the surface of a mast cell, a special cell found in everybody that is filled with chemical mediators, which turn out to be important in inflammation, especially allergic inflammation. When the allergen comes into the body again (e.g., in the nose, bronchial tubes, GI tract), the antibody made against it is activated, which leads to the mast cell it is "sitting on" releasing potent molecules or mediators that cause tissues to become inflamed. This inflammation and other actions resulting from the mediators are what cause the various problems and symptoms seen in asthma, hay fever, anaphylaxis, food allergy, insect sting allergy, and medication (e.g., antibiotic) allergy.

Since mast cells are concentrated in the airways, lining of the gastrointestinal tract, and skin, allergic reactions have their greatest effects on these parts of the body. Allergic responses vary greatly depending on the part of the body that is involved, and

WHAT HAPPENS DURING AN ALLERGIC REACTION

1. The allergen enters the body; it may be inhaled (pollen, dust mite, animal dander, viruses), swallowed (penicillin and other medications, certain food substances), injected (bee venom, penicillin), or come into direct contact with the skin or eyes.
2. The immune system recognizes the substance as foreign and responds by producing an antibody called immunoglobulin E, or IgE. This antibody molecule is programmed to remember and act against the specific allergen.
3. The IgE molecules latch on to the surfaces of mast cells, which help promote inflammation to fight off infection. Mast cells are normally abundant in the connective tissue of the skin, upper airways and lungs, and lining of the stomach and intestines. A person will not experience an allergic reaction to this initial exposure, but if he or she is vulnerable to allergies, the antibodies will stay on the alert for future encounters with the allergen.
4. If, at some future time, the allergen again enters the body, it is drawn to and links up with the IgE molecules on the mast cells.
5. When the allergen binds to the IgE molecule, tiny granules inside the mast cells are released. These granules contain inflammatory substances, especially histamine, but also various other biologically active molecules. It is these substances that cause the inflammation, swelling, itching, and other symptoms of an allergic response.

differ from one person to another and even within one person over time. Some people just suffer from hay fever, others from asthma, and yet others have combinations of different allergy manifestations or conditions (see box, *Symptoms Associated with*

Allergies, p. 7). The reason for this variety of symptoms (manifestations) is unknown.

Sometimes it takes years of exposure to an allergen before symptoms appear. Take, for example, the case of Reggie Allen. Over the years, he had been given penicillin several times for childhood infections. When he was in college, he developed a severe strep throat and was given an injection of penicillin. Within hours, Reggie developed extensive hives (itchy welts) and his entire arm was swollen. Antihistamines calmed this allergic reaction, and Reggie was warned that in the future he should wear a medical identification tag to let health-care workers know that he was hypersensitive to penicillin. Further use of the medication might result in an even more severe reaction called anaphylaxis, which can be fatal (see box, *Warning*, below).

This, of course, is an extreme example. Most allergies can be kept in check by a combination of identifying and avoiding potential allergens, together with the use of various medications.

WHO'S AT RISK?

Although allergies can develop at any age, they most commonly show up during childhood or early adulthood. A search of family

WARNING

Anaphylaxis—a rare but by far the most severe allergic reaction—is a life-threatening medical emergency that requires immediate treatment to prevent death. Symptoms usually occur immediately after exposure, but may be delayed for minutes to hours. Signs and symptoms include widespread swelling, agitation and anxiety, difficulty breathing due to swelling of the mouth and throat, wheezing, racing or pounding heart, convulsions, and loss of consciousness. For a more detailed discussion of anaphylaxis, see Chapter 6, "Killer Allergies: Anaphylaxis."

Symptoms Associated with Allergies

Eyes, Ears, Nose, and Mouth
- Red, teary, and/or itchy eyes
- Puffiness around the eyes
- Sneezing
- Runny nose
- Itchy nose, nose rubbing
- Postnasal drip
- Nasal swelling and congestion
- Itchy ear canals
- Itching of the mouth and throat

Lungs
- Hacking dry cough or cough that produces clear mucus
- Wheezing (noisy breathing)
- Feeling of tightness in the chest
- Low exercise tolerance
- Gasping for air; shortness of breath

Skin
- Eczema (patches of itchy, red skin rash)
- Hives (welts)

Intestines
- Cramps and intestinal discomfort
- Diarrhea
- Nausea and/or vomiting

Miscellaneous
- Headache
- Feelings of restlessness, irritability
- Excessive fatigue

medical histories of a child with allergies will usually turn up a close relative who also has allergies. If one parent has allergies, there is a 25 percent chance that a child will also have allergies. The risk is much higher if both parents are allergic. But the child will not necessarily be allergic to the same substances as the parents, or always show the same type of allergy manifestation (for example, hay fever or asthma or eczema).

WHEN TO SUSPECT AN ALLERGY

As indicated by the cases reported at the beginning of this chapter, allergies take many forms. Some are easy to identify by the pattern of symptoms that invariably follows exposure to a particular substance. But others are more subtle and may masquerade as other conditions. Here are some common clues that should lead you to suspect your child may have an allergy.

- Patches of bumps or of itchy, red skin that "weeps," or oozes clear fluid, and forms a crust (see Chapter 3, "Skin Allergies").
- Development of hives, intensely itchy skin eruptions that usually last for a few hours and move from one part of the body to another (see Chapter 3, "Skin Allergies," and Chapter 5, "Food Allergies").
- Repeated or chronic coldlike symptoms, such as a runny nose, nasal stuffiness, sneezing, and throat clearing, that last more than a week or two, or develop at about the same time every year (see Chapter 4, "Hay Fever").
- Nose rubbing, sniffling, snorting, sneezing.
- Itchy, runny eyes.
- Itching or tingling sensations in the mouth and throat (see Chapter 5, "Food Allergies").
- Coughing, wheezing, difficulty breathing, and other respiratory symptoms (see Chapter 8, "An Overview of Asthma").
- Unexplained bouts of diarrhea, abdominal cramps, and other intestinal symptoms.

WHERE DOES ASTHMA FIT IN?

Although allergies and asthma often go together, they are actually two different conditions. In simple terms, asthma is a chronic condition originating in the lungs, whereas allergies originate in the immune system. Many different substances and circumstances can trigger an asthma attack—exercise, exposure to cold air, a viral infection, air pollution, noxious fumes, tobacco smoke, and, for many asthma sufferers, a host of allergens. In fact, about 80 percent of children with asthma also have allergies and, for them, allergens are often the most common asthma triggers. Here are a few real-life examples of how asthma can appear.

Ed and Mary Alice both suffer from allergies—Ed is very allergic to cats, ragweed pollen, and dust mites, while hay fever makes summer a misery for Mary Alice. At first, they thought that their son Danny had escaped his parents' allergies. He didn't have a trace of eczema or unusual sneezing, sniffling, and other allergy symptoms, even when he played with a neighbor's cat. At about age 3, however, Danny developed a persistent cough that seemed to worsen at night. Then Danny caught a bad cold and, just when he seemed to be recovering nicely, he began wheezing and breathing with great difficulty. Mary Alice immediately called her pediatrician, who told her to bring Danny to the emergency department. There doctors quickly determined that Danny was having an attack of asthma. Prompt treatment brought the attack under control, but that episode marked the beginning of a long struggle to keep Danny's asthma in check.

Michelle's story is quite different. Neither of her parents has allergies and there is no family history of asthma on either side. When Michelle was about 2 years old, her parents noticed that she wheezed and coughed a lot. They thought the problem was an enlarged adenoid, but were shocked when their pediatrician told them Michelle had asthma.

Nine-year-old Rodney, a budding soccer player, seemed to live for the sport. But his junior league coach was concerned about the shortness of breath that often forced a very frustrated Rodney to take to the sidelines. The coach urged Rodney's parents to consult their pediatrician, who diagnosed the young athlete's problem as exercise-induced asthma.

These brief case histories illustrate just a few of the many ways in which asthma can manifest itself. But regardless of the manner of onset, what happens in the lungs is pretty much the same. The bronchi—the tubes that carry air in and out of the lungs—are abnormally hypersensitive. It turns out that everybody's bronchi are capable of becoming narrow, or constricted, possibly to protect the lungs against the entry of harmful substances. In asthma, the bronchi are overly sensitive and tighten up in the presence of normally harmless substances. Many doctors describe asthmatic bronchi as "twitchy."

But there's another side to asthma. The hypersensitive bronchi become inflamed, which results in internal swelling and increased production of mucus. This inflammation, in turn, is important in making the bronchi twitchy. When bronchi develop low-grade, long-standing inflammation, the result is chronic asthma. Tightening of the bronchi, along with the inflammation and swelling, makes it doubly difficult to breathe. The child with this condition may complain of a tight feeling in the chest, have a deep cough, or develop wheezing (a whistling noise) from the lungs.

Use of an inhaled bronchodilator—medication that relaxes the muscles controlling the bronchi—can usually stop an asthma attack. Other medications are given to stop the inflammation. Very often, medications are used daily, even when the asthma seems to be quiet, to calm the twitchy bronchi and control inflammation. The proper use of asthma medications, coupled with lifestyle changes that come from identifying and avoiding as many asthma triggers as possible, is the key to successful asthma control. Unfortunately, this is often easier said than done. For a more detailed discussion of all aspects of asthma, see Chapters 8 to 13.

CHAPTER 2

Establishing the Diagnosis

S even-year-old Johnny has been diagnosed with recurrent bronchitis since he was only a few months old. In a typical episode, Johnny starts coughing, then wheezing, and finally, his chest becomes congested and he has trouble breathing. At the clinic where his family receives medical care, the doctors routinely prescribe an antibiotic to clear up the bacterial infection they believe is causing the bronchitis. Johnny also gets a liquid medication to open up the airways, relieve the cough, and make it easier to breathe. Johnny asks his mother for a dose of this "cough medicine" almost every day.

Johnny's bronchitis attacks have become more frequent and severe in the three years since he started school. His mother also notices that Johnny starts wheezing whenever he runs or plays hard. Johnny often misses school because of his chest problems and bronchitis.

During the intervals when Johnny isn't coughing, wheezing,

*O*ne common pattern *of allergy-related problems starts in infancy with eczema and food allergy. Next follows a phase often marked by recurrent infections of the ears, throat, and sinuses with upper respiratory symptoms. Finally, obvious—or not so obvious—symptoms of hay fever and/or asthma may appear.*

and having breathing problems, he has a nonstop runny nose, his eyes and nose are itchy, and he complains that his ears are blocked. At Johnny's last clinic visit, the doctor sent him for X rays, which showed that he had sinusitis, an inflammation of the sinuses—air spaces in the bones of the face that connect with the nasal passages. This condition is often, but not always, caused by a bacterial infection. After yet another course of antibiotic treatment, his symptoms improved a little but did not completely go away.

For years, Johnny's mother has told herself that the youngster will grow out of his symptoms but, instead, they are getting worse. On learning that both parents have hay fever and that Johnny's mother has asthma, the clinic doctor reviews the boy's medical records and refers him for a complete evaluation for probable asthma and allergies.

— ❖ —

FIRST, THE HISTORY...

Diagnosis follows an orderly process that starts with a careful medical history. Your pediatrician will ask a lot of questions about your child's symptoms and medical background, and about your family's medical history as well.

- Does your child cough, wheeze, or get extra short of breath when she's running or playing hard?
- Does your child cough a lot? Is the coughing worse at night? Is she wheezing? Does she have trouble breathing? Does her chest feel tight sometimes?
- What happens when she laughs or becomes upset?
- Does your child sneeze frequently? Does she rub her nose often? Does she blow her nose or wipe it a lot? Is the nasal discharge clear and runny? (A clear discharge is typical of allergic rhinitis, also called hay fever, the most common form of allergy; see box, *Allergic Rhinitis and Asthma*, p. 15.) Or is it thick and greenish or yellowish? (A yellow or green color suggests that your child may have an infection, possibly in addition to allergy symptoms.)

SYMPTOMS: ALL IN THE TIMING

Allergy symptoms that come and go with the seasons may be caused by seasonal plants and crops. Coughing, sneezing, or other chest and nose symptoms that get much better when your child is away from home may indicate that your child is sensitive to substances normally found indoors, such as pets. By contrast, symptoms that always clear up on weekends and school vacations suggest that there may be a problem with something in the environment at school.

Coughing at night with hoarseness and frequent throat clearing may be caused by postnasal drip due to allergic rhinitis or sinusitis. But coughing, wheezing, and related symptoms that get worse at night may also raise suspicions about asthma, because asthma symptoms are often worse at night. Your pediatrician may perform tests for exercise-induced asthma if your child frequently coughs and/or wheezes when running or playing energetically.

- Are her eyes itchy and watery?
- Does she have more than her share of colds? Do they last longer than a week?
- Does she ever have a rash or itchy bumps on the skin?
- How often does she have symptoms? How long do they last?
- Do particular events seem to bring on symptoms, or make them better or worse?
- Have the symptoms ever gotten better after your child has taken medicine? What kind of medication helped?

Your pediatrician will ask whether your child's symptoms often appear during a particular season of the year, at a certain location, or when your child is around animals, such as cats. He or she will also ask whether symptoms come on after your child has eaten a particular food.

Your pediatrician will ask whether other members of the family have hay fever, asthma, or eczema, because allergy and asthma run in families (see box, *Allergies Tend to Run in Families*, below). However, even if you can't recall a single relative who sneezes and wheezes, your doctor will not discount allergy and asthma in your child because, like many disorders, they can appear out of the blue.

Parents sometimes try over-the-counter medications before asking their pediatricians about a persistent cough, a rash, or respiratory symptoms. Although it's recommended that you talk to

ALLERGIES TEND TO RUN IN FAMILIES

Many types of allergy problems, including hay fever, asthma, and eczema, tend to run in families. If both parents have allergies, each child has about a 60 to 70 percent chance of being allergic.

However, allergic responses to insect venom, medications, and latex are the exceptions to the rule. Having a parent with one of these allergies does not increase the chance that a child will be allergic.

your pediatrician before giving medications to your child, it's helpful to tell the doctor whether a medication had any effect, because this can give clues about the possible cause of symptoms. For example, if a runny nose and itchiness bothered your child less and she stopped sneezing for a while after taking an antihistamine, chances are she has an allergy and not an infection. Conversely, if her coughing and wheezing did not change after she took a dose of over-the-counter cough syrup, your pediatrician may decide to test for asthma before looking for other underlying conditions.

THEN, THE PHYSICAL EXAMINATION...

Your child's weight and height will be measured and compared with her records to make sure she is growing and gaining weight at a satisfactory rate. (Severe asthma can sometimes interfere with growth.) Your pediatrician will note whether your child is breathing through the mouth because of a stuffed-up nose. The doctor

ALLERGIC RHINITIS AND ASTHMA

The word "rhinitis" means inflammation of the membranes lining the nose. Typical symptoms include a runny nasal discharge, stuffiness, and sneezing many times in a row. If allergies are the cause, the condition is called allergic rhinitis and, in addition to the other symptoms, the nose is often itchy. Pollens (grasses, trees, and weeds) are common culprits. Seasonal allergic rhinitis is also known as "hay fever," even though it's not caused by hay and doesn't involve fever.

Allergic rhinitis stops a person from breathing through the nose, with its natural filters and air-warming system. Those with allergic rhinitis have an increased risk of asthma. A possible reason is that open-mouth breathing lets larger amounts of asthma triggers pass into the airways along with cooler, drier air, both of which can trigger asthma attacks, bringing on wheezing, coughing, and gasping for breath.

will also look for "allergic shiners," bruiselike discolorations around the eyes that are frequently signs of chronic nasal blockage. These signs may indicate that your child has allergic rhinitis or allergic conjunctivitis.

A youngster whose nose is always running may unconsciously make a gesture that has been termed the "allergic salute"—a quick upward swipe to the nose. By pushing the nose upward dozens of times a day, some children actually develop a permanent crease across the nose where the pliable cartilage meets the bony bridge. Your pediatrician will look inside your child's nose to see if the lining is swollen and either pale (typical of allergies) or unusually red (often seen with infection). He or she will also note the color of the mucus, since discharge due to allergies is normally clear or white.

Your doctor will look for redness due to allergic inflammation in the whites of your child's eyes, and for bumps on the lining of the eyelids, which are also signs of allergies. Examination of the chest may show an unusual barrel shape, which is sometimes a sign of asthma. Using the stethoscope, your doctor will listen for wheezes and other unusual sounds that may be heard in asthma. He or she will look over your child's skin for rashes, particularly dry, scratched-over patches near the joints, which can indicate eczema.

Finally, the Tests

BLOOD TESTS. Blood tests may be ordered—first, for an indication of your child's general health, and second, to count the numbers of eosinophils, a type of white blood cell involved in allergic responses. An unusually high eosinophil count points to possible allergies.

Your pediatrician may also order a total allergy antibody test, called an IgE level (see p. 4). The total IgE level does not detect specific allergies. However, if the total IgE level is higher than normal, there's a strong possibility that your child has allergies. Skin testing or a radioallergosorbent blood test (RAST, see p. 19) needs to be done to identify what triggers the allergies (see following sections). Your pediatrician may refer you to a pediatric allergist for these tests.

SKIN TESTS. Skin tests, first developed almost a century ago, are still the mainstay of allergy testing. They are easy to do, give fast results, and are relatively inexpensive, which makes them the best way to start looking for specific allergies.

In "scratch" skin tests, drops of allergen extracts—for example, pollens, dust mites, molds, animal danders, and foods, among others—are allowed to seep through shallow scratches made in the patient's skin. The tests can also be performed by the deeper, intradermal technique, in which the extracts are injected under the skin. There are pros and cons to both testing methods. Scratch tests are painless and very easy to do. They are somewhat less sensitive than intradermal tests; they are also less likely to

SKIN TESTS MUST BE DONE BY AN EXPERIENCED PHYSICIAN

Although a positive result to scratch or intradermal skin testing strongly suggests that your child has formed IgE antibodies against a specific allergen, it does not follow that he will develop allergy symptoms when exposed to that particular allergen in the environment. As a rule, the bigger the skin-test reaction, the higher the chances are that your child is allergic and will sneeze, itch, or break out in a rash. However, in some cases the skin reaction is trivial while the symptoms are overwhelming, and vice versa. Further, even though your child may have diminished symptoms as he gets older, the skin-test result can remain positive. It is important that tests be conducted, and results interpreted, by someone trained and experienced in allergy skin testing.

cause a severe reaction in someone who is highly allergic. The intradermal tests, which let the allergen extracts penetrate deeper into the skin, are highly sensitive, but they can occasionally result in false positive reactions, indicating allergies where none exist. Your physician may decide to start with scratch tests, then go on to intradermal testing if further information is needed. Before testing, your doctor will ask you not to give your child any anti-

Many parents and children are afraid of having allergy skin testing because they've heard false reports that it is painful and upsetting. Scratch tests, the form of testing most often used in children, are mostly painless, because they are done on the surface of the skin, where there aren't any nerve endings to register pain. Further, new test devices are available, which can do up to eight tests at a time and allow scratch testing to be done very quickly and without injury. The intradermal technique uses a very fine needle to penetrate the surface of the skin. It is "felt" a little more than scratch testing, but is still not very painful.

Many people also falsely believe that children have to reach a certain age before they can be tested. In fact, age is no barrier to skin testing; positive results can be obtained at any age. For example, in infants and toddlers who have eczema and suspected food allergy, skin tests often reveal sensitivity to milk or egg. Once parents have this information, they can keep the foods out of their child's diet to control allergy symptoms.

Finally, experienced doctors and nurses perform allergy testing on a daily basis. They know how to take away fears and put children—and parents—at their ease.

histamines for 48 to 72 hours, as they will interfere with the results of the tests.

If your child has formed specific IgE antibodies through earlier exposure to one of the substances being tested, the skin will redden and swell into a disk that looks like a mosquito bite around the puncture site. This skin reaction usually comes on within 15 minutes after the test extracts are applied, peaks between 15 and 30 minutes, and then gradually clears up.

Allergy skin testing is safe and relatively painless if conducted properly by an experienced physician or clinic. The skin where the tests were done may feel itchy for a few hours. However, if your child develops severe itching, wheezing, light-headedness, or shortness of breath after you get home, call your doctor at once or take your child to the nearest emergency department.

RADIOALLERGOSORBENT TEST (RAST). Instead of skin tests, your pediatrician or allergy specialist may order a radioallergosorbent blood test, called RAST, to identify specific allergies. The RAST is especially useful if skin tests cannot be done because, for instance, a child has eczema over much of his body, or cannot be taken off medication that interferes with skin testing. A RAST shows up specific sensitivities, as skin tests do, but does so by detecting the presence of allergy antibodies circulating in the blood. If antibodies are in the blood, it usually means that the same antibodies are also in other tissues. The method is not quite as versatile as skin testing, because certain extracts are not available for RAST testing. For example, a RAST cannot be used to detect sensitivity to medications and is rarely used to detect insect venom allergy. However, a RAST is adaptable and sensitive enough to detect a wide range of allergies. The procedure costs more per test than skin testing. It takes only a few minutes of the patient's time to draw a blood sample and there is no risk of any allergic reaction. The RAST results take from 5 to 14 days, whereas skin test results are available immediately.

X RAYS AND IMAGING TESTS. While sometimes useful, X rays are not essential for diagnosing asthma or allergies. In fact, people with asthma usually have normal chest X rays. However, chest X rays are sometimes done to make sure children do not have other conditions that can mimic asthma.

Sinus infection can produce symptoms similar to those of respiratory allergies, and children who have respiratory allergies are prone to sinus infections. Your pediatrician may order an imaging test to see if your child simply has a prolonged or recurrent infection, or whether a sinus infection is complicating his allergies. An imaging test can be done the old-fashioned way, with an X ray of the head, or it can be performed by computerized tomography

(CT). A CT scan is more sensitive than an X ray and shows finer details of the anatomy of the sinuses, which can help your pediatrician decide on the best way to treat your child's sinus problem.

Finally, imaging tests can sometimes help your pediatrician identify the reason that your child snores or has a permanently stuffed-up nose. An X ray of the upper neck area can show if the stuffiness is caused by enlargement of the adenoid tissue, which sits in the upper throat just behind the nose.

LUNG-FUNCTION TESTS. If your child has symptoms indicating possible asthma, your pediatrician may perform tests to evaluate the lung function. Lung-function tests are performed in your pediatrician's office or a pulmonary function laboratory where special equipment is available. An instrument called a spirometer is used to measure how much air your child can breathe out, as well

ASTHMA SCREENING

The American College of Asthma, Allergy and Immunology conducts an annual Nationwide Asthma Screening Program for children and adults in more than 200 communities. With the support of the Asthma and Allergy Foundation of America and the Allergy and Asthma Network/Mothers of Asthmatics, this free program screened approximately 10,000 people in 1998, its third year of operation. To find out where screening is available, visit www.allergy.mcg.edu, or write Asthma Screening Program, 35 East Wacker Drive, Suite 1254, Chicago, IL 60601.

as how fast the air flows. The pediatrician will place a clip over your child's nose to prevent air escaping from the nostrils. He or she will then ask your child to perform breathing maneuvers into a mouthpiece attached to a pulmonary function monitor. The maneuvers aren't difficult or painful. All your child has to do is take a deep breath, then breathe out forcefully through the mouthpiece. Instead of using a spirometer, the doctor may ask your child to blow into a simpler device called a peak flow meter (see p. 130). Your pediatrician usually performs the lung-function test at least three times to make sure results are consistent.

If lung testing shows that your child cannot blow air out fast enough, your pediatrician may perform further tests for asthma. He or she may give your child a dose of bronchodilator medication to see if there is a change in the air flow. If the air flow is normal or improved after the medication, the result strongly suggests that asthma is present.

FOOD DIARY. If your pediatrician suspects that your child has a food allergy, he or she may ask you to keep a food diary for several weeks. Use the diary to write down every single food your child eats and any symptoms that follow within minutes to a few hours after a particular meal or snack.

The food diary may be used together with an elimination diet. Your pediatrician will give you a list of foods to keep out of your child's diet for a certain period. You may then be instructed to reintroduce each food one at a time at intervals of several days, using the diary to note any symptoms that recur or appear for the first time. This method, called food avoidance and rechallenge, may help to establish whether a specific food allergy is present.

If your pediatrician has any concerns about the possibility of a life-threatening anaphylactic reaction (see p. 6 and Chapter 6, "Killer Allergies: Anaphylaxis"), you will be instructed not to reintroduce the suspect food at home. Instead, your pediatrician may perform a food-challenge test, if required, in the clinic setting where emergency care is available. However, if your child's history is suspicious, such a challenge may be too dangerous and will not be done.

A food challenge is sometimes done to double-check the results of skin testing or a RAST, or when the food avoidance and rechallenge method has not provided enough information. Under close observation in the pediatrician's or allergy specialist's office, your child will be asked to swallow a very small amount of the suspect food, possibly in the form of a gelatin capsule. If there is an allergy, symptoms will appear anywhere from 5 to 60 minutes after the challenge.

SWEAT TEST. Cystic fibrosis is an inherited disorder that involves many body systems. It causes symptoms in the respiratory and digestive tracts that can mimic those of asthma and allergies. A child with cystic fibrosis may have asthma and/or allergies, as well. Your pediatrician may order tests to measure the levels of certain minerals in your child's sweat. If the results indicate cystic fibrosis, further tests will be done to confirm the diagnosis.

What Happens Next?

After making an initial diagnosis of allergy on the basis of the history and symptoms, and performing skin tests and/or a RAST, your child's pediatrician or allergy specialist will advise on the best course of treatment. If your child's symptoms don't improve after a trial of treatment, further tests may be warranted.

Part II

*Recognizing and Dealing
with Allergies*

CHAPTER 3

Skin Allergies

When Christine was 6 months old, her mother weaned her from breastmilk to a cow's-milk-based formula. Christine had occasionally spat up, but now she started vomiting after meals. At the same time, a dry, crusty rash appeared on her cheeks, then spread behind her ears, onto her neck, and over her arms and legs. Christine, normally a happy infant, seemed irritable with the rash. Her mother often found Christine rubbing her face against the sheets even while she slept, which made the rash worse. The vomiting stopped when Christine's pediatrician switched her to a low-allergenic formula made with hydrolyzed protein. He explained that Christine's rash was atopic dermatitis, commonly called eczema, often an early sign of allergy problems. The doctor prescribed a low-

The most common chronic inflammatory skin condition in children is eczema, also called atopic dermatitis. Although not strictly an allergic disorder, eczema in young children has many of the hallmarks of allergies and is often a harbinger of hay fever and asthma. The rate of eczema, like that of asthma, is increasing throughout the world. Where asthma is rare, the rate of eczema is also low.

DIAPER RASH IS NOT ECZEMA

If your baby has a crusty rash in the diaper area, consult your pediatrician. Treatment may be required to soothe the irritation and clear up an infection. Protect against diaper rash with a zinc oxide cream. Avoid using commercial wet wipes, which may contain irritating compounds. Clean your baby with plain warm water.

strength cortisone cream and a sedating antihistamine to be given at bedtime. Regular use of these medications helped keep the rash under control.

The rash became worse after Christine had her first fried egg, at around age 1. She also broke out in hives. After this, her parents were careful to keep eggs out of her diet, but occasionally a dish made with a small amount of egg, such as noodles, slipped past them. Christine's eczema always flared up right after she ate a food containing egg.

By Christine's third birthday, her skin rash was gradually getting better, but her mother called their pediatrician when Christine started wheezing during a cold, as the doctor had warned she might. Even after her cold cleared up, Christine had a nonstop runny, stuffed-up nose.

When Christine was ready for kindergarten at age 5, her eczema was completely gone. However, her pediatrician had di-

ECZEMA: NOT QUITE ALLERGY?

Eczema has some puzzling features that don't fit neatly into the pattern we recognize as allergy. For example, children with eczema usually have high blood levels of IgE, the antibody involved in allergic reactions. However, their allergy skin tests don't always reveal evidence of allergy or, if they do, the substances in question are often not important factors in the eczema.

agnosed chronic asthma and hay fever. These conditions were kept under control with regular use of medications.

— ❖ —

For many parents, the first sign that they should be on the watch for, in allergies of all kinds, is a single patch of raised white bumps, or a dry, red, crusty rash that starts on their baby's cheeks and spreads over most of the face and body. The "look" of eczema varies: Although it can appear weepy, it is more commonly dry, scaly, or crusty. The rash is intensely itchy—a hallmark of eczema. In fact, itching often sets in before a rash appears. The discomfort may change the baby's mood; an infant who was formerly content may become continually irritable.

NOT YOUR USUAL REACTION

In eczema, the skin has an unusual reaction to nonallergenic contacts as well as allergens. For example, if you lightly run the back of your thumbnail down the inside of your forearm, within seconds you will see a red streak. Perform the same test on the arm of your child with eczema and you may see a red streak that is rapidly replaced by a white one. This is called white dermographism.

The patches of skin affected by eczema also cool down and warm up at different rates from normal skin, especially in the folds of the body—inside the elbows, neck, and armpits.

Eczema affects between 5 and 10 percent of children, and usually—but not always—disappears before adulthood. However, in most cases, as children outgrow eczema they develop typical symptoms of respiratory allergy, such as hay fever (see Chapter 4) or asthma (see Chapters 8 to 13). About 75 percent of children with eczema develop another form of allergy at some point. Children tend to develop asthma at an earlier age if they start out

PSORIASIS: NOT ECZEMA, NOT ALLERGY

A school-age child may develop a rash of red lumps that spread and join up to form irregular patches, most often on the elbows, knees, and scalp, or around the navel. Eventually, the patches become covered with thick white scales. As the child scratches the scales, pinpoints of bleeding will appear on the new skin underneath.

These patches are typical of psoriasis. Unlike eczema, psoriasis is not an allergic condition. Frequently, there is a family history of psoriasis, and the child may have had unusually extensive cradle cap in infancy or dandruff in the toddler and preschool years. The condition occurs in both sexes, but is more common in girls. Attacks of psoriasis are often linked to periods of emotional stress, such as exam time at school. In some children, psoriasis may follow a strep throat.

Do not try to remove the scales or treat the condition with over-the-counter remedies. If your pediatrician diagnoses psoriasis, your child may be referred to a dermatologist.

with eczema. Interestingly, about 20 percent of all patients with eczema never have any sign of allergies and they usually do not have a family history of allergy problems.

Most children with eczema develop symptoms in their first 1 to 2 years of life, and almost all before age 5. The pattern of symptoms differs according to children's ages. In infants and young children, the rash generally appears on the face (except around the nose), scalp, abdomen, arms, and legs. It may cover the trunk and back, but almost never spreads to the diaper area (see box, *Diaper Rash Is Not Eczema,* p. 25). Before 4 to 6 months of age, infants don't have the muscular coordination to scratch the itch. Instead, they try to ease the intense discomfort by rubbing their faces against the bedclothes or the sides of their cribs. This breaks the skin surface, causing weeping and crusting, and the baby becomes even more uncomfortable, especially if the broken skin becomes infected. In older children, the eczema rash is usually confined to the skin folds, such as the creases of the elbows, knees, and neck. Occasionally, the rash covers the wrists, hands, ankles, and feet (but not the palms and soles), while the rest of the body may remain clear.

Over time and with constant scratching, the eczematous skin can become dry, darker, and thickened, and the normal surface lines are deeper. These changes are called "lichenification."

A CRUSTY RASH MAY BE IMPETIGO

The rash of eczema can sometimes break, weep, and form a crusty scab. But if you see large, spreading blisters with reddening, warmth, and puffy swelling, or oozing and crust formation, your child may have impetigo. This is a skin infection caused by streptococcus or staphylococcus bacteria. Call your pediatrician; if your child has impetigo, antibiotic treatment is required to clear up the condition and prevent it from spreading to others.

IDENTIFYING TRIGGERS

Your pediatrician considers many factors in looking for the cause of eczema. Researchers estimate that food allergy plays a role in about 25 percent of cases of eczema in young children. The protein in egg white is the most common food allergy trigger after infancy. However, the atypical nature of eczema can make it difficult to pinpoint a specific food sensitivity. Allergy skin testing or a RAST can sometimes be helpful. Alternatively, your pediatrician may simply review your child's history, then suggest that you either withhold a suspect food or try a low-allergenic diet for 7 to 10 days to see if symptoms improve. If you don't see a change for the better after 10 to 14 days, foods probably don't play a role in your child's skin troubles. You should try these measures only on your pediatrician's advice, to make sure that your child is getting the nutrients she needs. For example, if your pediatrician advises you to keep milk and dairy foods out of the diet, he or she may recommend alternative sources of calcium and vitamins.

Although children with eczema may develop respiratory allergies later on, sensitivity to airborne allergens such as pollens and molds does not seem to be an important trigger for eczema. However, the rash may be brought on or worsened by contact with dust mites and animal danders.

The rash of eczema can be aggravated by many nonallergenic environmental conditions, such as wide swings in temperature or humidity, extremely dry air, scratchy or tight clothing, and sweating. Many children with eczema cannot tolerate wool next to their skin. Skin symptoms, especially scratching, sometimes get worse when a youngster is overtired, nervous, or emotionally upset.

In getting to the source of your child's eczema, your pediatrician will look for other possible causes of an itchy, scaling rash. In young infants, cradle cap, or seborrheic dermatitis, can resemble eczema. However, cradle cap usually appears before 6 weeks of age and does not make the baby itchy and irritable. Parasites, such as lice and scabies, and irritating substances can produce similar symptoms, but the distribution of the rash is usually different from the characteristic pattern of eczema. These conditions usually clear up quite rapidly with treatment. Extremely severe eczema may be a sign that an infant has a severe underlying condition (such as an immune deficiency) that should be investigated.

MANAGING ECZEMA

In addition to the dietary approaches mentioned earlier, your pediatrician can recommend measures to help clear up the rash and itching, and reduce exposure to possible triggers of eczema (for a detailed discussion of treatment, see Chapter 7). Antihistamine medication may be prescribed to relieve the itching and help break the itch-scratch cycle (which leads to more itching, scratching, and possibly infection). Your pediatrician may advise giving the medication at night; some antihistamines have the side effect of mild drowsiness, which can help the child sleep better and suppress the urge to scratch during sleep. Long-sleeved sleepwear may also help to prevent nighttime scratching.

A cortisone medication will be prescribed to reduce inflammation. This usually needs to be applied regularly (once or twice a day) to control the rash. Cortisone creams and ointments are

Choose Soaps and Detergents with Care

Soaps containing perfumes and deodorants may be too harsh for children's sensitive skin. Many pediatricians recommend nonsoap cleansing lotions for infants and neutral, unperfumed, full-fat soaps or glycerin soaps for toddlers and older children. Children who cannot tolerate woolen clothing next to the skin may also be hypersensitive to lanolin-based soaps and lotions.

Use laundry products that are free of dyes and perfumes, and double-rinse clothes, towels, and bedding. If you have concerns about any personal care product, don't use it on your child.

available in various strengths. Some are too strong to be applied to the face and certain other parts of the body. These and all medications must be used exactly as prescribed to prevent side effects. A nonsedating antihistamine also can be used during the day when your child needs to stay alert for school.

Warm (never hot) showers may be preferable to baths. In addition, moisturizing baths in lukewarm water for 20 minutes add moisture to the epithelial layer and cleanse the skin by lowering the number of bacteria. Gently pat your child dry after the shower or bath to avoid irritating the skin with rubbing. Apply a moisturizer or lubricating cream to the whole body within 3 minutes, while the skin is still moist. This helps to keep the skin from drying out.

CLOTHING SHOULDN'T GET UNDER YOUR CHILD'S SKIN

Some synthetic fabrics, silk, and dyes and other chemicals used in manufacturing can irritate sensitive skin. Launder new clothes thoroughly before your child wears them. Look for T-shirts and underwear made of undyed cotton that your child can wear next to the skin. Cut off labels and turn undergarments inside out to keep scratchy seams and trimmings from irritating your child's skin. Use cotton sheets and blankets.

The more your child scratches, the greater the risk of the skin's becoming infected. An antibiotic given either by mouth or in the form of an ointment to rub on the skin may be necessary to clear up the infection. Antibiotic treatment may help to clear up the rash as well, since the staphylococcus bacteria that commonly cause skin infections also trigger eczema in some cases. Keep your child's fingernails clean and short to reduce the risk of injury from scratching and prevent contamination of open scratches.

If possible, install air-conditioning in your child's room to keep the temperature even. Call your pediatrician promptly if your child's rash gets worse or recurs despite treatment.

HIVES

Jeremy, 4 years old, has a bad cold and a bronchial infection, which keeps him awake with coughing through the night. His pediatrician prescribes amoxicillin, an antibiotic, to clear up the bronchial infection. Five days after the start of the cold, Jeremy breaks out in hives. His body is covered in the typical rash of large and small itchy welts. Believing that the hives are an allergic reaction to the antibiotic, the doctor stops the medication and prescribes a different antibiotic as well as an antihistamine to stop the itching and swelling, and the hives gradually disappear.

Jeremy has no problems until 6 months later, when he catches another cold and again develops hives. This time he's not taking an antibiotic. Antihistamine treatment helps, but the hives take about 2 weeks to disappear completely. During each bout of hives, the welts are especially numerous around Jeremy's waist and the tops of his thighs, where the elastic in his underwear presses on the skin. The results of allergy testing do not indicate sensitivity to amoxicillin or the related antibiotic, penicillin, which are common causes of allergy. And, according to the tests, Jeremy does not have any other allergies. After these early episodes, Jeremy never has another bout of hives.

At least 1 child in 5 has a bout of the itchy welts known as hives, or urticaria, at one time or another. Although there may well be a specific cause for the hives, it's not always possible to identify it before the rash burns itself out. Therefore, if your child has an isolated bout, your pediatrician will concentrate on relieving the annoying symptoms, rather than lose time in looking for the cause. However, if hives recur or become chronic—that is, an episode lasts longer than 6 weeks—it is worthwhile to look for the trigger factors so that preventive measures can be taken. However, in many cases, the cause of chronic hives is never found.

Hives are intensely itchy, raised welts that resemble mosquito bites or the rash caused by stinging nettles. The welts usually appear in clusters and may run together to form a single large, raised swelling. Whether isolated or joined up, individual welts usually disappear anywhere from 2 to 24 hours after first emerging. However, new hives promptly appear on another part of the body to begin the cycle over again.

Often, hives are accompanied by angioedema, a deeper, more

diffuse swelling that comes and goes with the same baffling unpredictability as the itchy welts. Hives appear most often on the trunk and limbs, but may pop up anywhere. In contrast, angioedema usually affects loose tissue, such as the cheeks, lips, tongue, and skin around the eyes, although it can appear on the limbs as well. Angioedema is not usually itchy, but may feel painful, burning, or simply "strange." The swellings of angioedema come and go, as hives do, and may occur whether hives are present or not.

HOME REMEDIES TO SOOTHE ITCHY SKIN

If your child prefers baths to showers, a couple of tablespoons of baking soda in tepid bathwater can soothe the itch of eczema or hives. Or tie a cup of oatmeal in cheesecloth and swish it through the lukewarm bathwater until the water looks a little cloudy. You can make a traditional skin remedy by soaking ½ cup of dried camomile (or 4 camomile tea bags) in a cup of hot water for 30 minutes, straining the liquid, and adding it to a tepid bath. Cold compresses (washcloths wrung out in cold water) may help to soothe an itch.

Creams and lotions made from the aloe plant are soothing to the skin. Commercial aloe products may contain only small amounts of the active extract. Instead, cut or tear the leaf of an aloe plant and rub the clear, gummy gel (not the yellow juice) on irritated skin.

Hives and angioedema can make your child extremely uncomfortable. Facial distortions caused by angioedema, in particular, can be quite frightening. Although distressing, these conditions are not usually serious. Both can be triggered by any substance to which a child is allergic. Foods (e.g., eggs, milk, peanuts, tree nuts) and medications, especially antibiotics, are the most frequent allergic causes. Often, a definite cause or trigger for hives is never identified. Eggs, peanuts, and tree nuts are common food triggers for hives in children. Children may suffer hives and angioedema during an otherwise mild viral infection. In rare cases, environmental factors such as exposure to cold or heat may cause hives or swelling. Usually, the symptoms go away by themselves and no treatment is required. However, if symptoms persist, call your pediatrician.

If you are certain there's a link between your child's hives and/or angioedema and a particular food, make every effort to keep it out of the diet. In the unlikely event that the food is an important source of nutrients, it's almost always possible to find a nonallergenic substitute that provides similar nutritional value.

Hives are sometimes produced or made worse by pressure, such as from tight clothes. If your child has a rash or itching along pressure lines from clothing, make sure he has comfortable, loose-fitting underwear and outerwear, including socks, belts, and shoes. Some children are vulnerable to hives and other skin troubles when they are feeling unusual emotional pressure, such as during exam time or a period of family stress.

Your pediatrician may prescribe antihistamine treatment for hives. In most cases, treatment is required for just a short while, but sometimes antihistamines are needed daily for weeks to keep hives suppressed. Hives often go away as mysteriously as they came. Depending on your child's history and the results of allergy testing, dietary and other measures may be recommended to prevent future episodes. (For details of treatment, see Chapter 7.)

CHAPTER 4

Hay Fever
(Allergic Rhinitis)

M ary is worried about starting first grade this fall. Her nose runs all the time with a clear, watery liquid, and she always needs to be near the tissue box. Last year in kindergarten, other children made fun of Mary because she wiped her nose so often and was constantly sniffing, making noises, and rubbing her nose. Even the teacher frequently asked if Mary had a cold.

When Mary was younger, she had a constant rash, which her pediatrician diagnosed as eczema. The skin condition and other symptoms, which were caused by a milk allergy, are much better now. However, about the time Mary's rash improved, she started having a runny, itchy nose. Mary's mother buys an over-the-counter antihistamine, which helps relieve the symptoms, but it makes Mary sleepy. Sometimes she even falls asleep in class if she takes the medication be-

These are the typical symptoms and signs of allergic rhinitis, a condition commonly known as hay fever and often recognized as "allergies."

- *Sneezing many times in a row.*
- *Blocked-up nose with a streaming, clear discharge.*
- *Itching of the eyes, nose, inside the ears, and in the roof of the mouth.*
- *Having to stay near the tissue box.*

fore school. Mary's father understands her problems because he has hay fever, with a nose that is constantly runny and itchy during pollen season and at other times when his allergies bother him. He has also noticed that Mary wheezes when she has a cold and tends to cough whenever she runs. He knows these can be symptoms of asthma, because when he was young he had asthma along with his hay fever, and hopes that Mary doesn't develop asthma as well. Mary's parents have made an appointment with their pediatrician for an evaluation of all Mary's symptoms. In particular, her father wants to talk to their pediatrician about possible treatments, as he has heard that new therapies for children's allergies are a big improvement over the medications that were available when he was growing up.

Hay fever (which is actually misnamed, since the symptoms are not caused by hay and don't include fever) typically starts in the early school years, but it can occur as early as the second year of life. A child is more likely to develop hay fever if his parents and other family members also have allergies. The condition is about twice as common in boys than it is in girls. In children, hay fever may follow an early period marked by eczema and other symptoms caused by food sensitivity (see Chapter 3, "Skin Allergies"). In many cases, sneezing, nonstop runny nose, and itchy eyes set in just as the recurrent skin rash and itching of eczema start to fade.

A family history of allergies is by far the most important key to the development of hay fever, especially when the symptoms appear during childhood. However, the rate of hay fever, like that of asthma, appears to be increasing all over the world. This may be because environmental conditions bring out symptoms in people who have inherited tendencies to allergic disorders.

IT'S THAT TIME AGAIN

You may have come to dread a particular time of the year—usually spring or fall—because with the regularity of clockwork, that's when your child's eyes, mouth, and ears start to itch, he sneezes many times in a row several times a day—some doctors describe it as "machine-gun sneezing"—and his nose is stuffed up and runs with a watery discharge from morning to night. In such cases, symptoms are most often triggered by allergies to pollens and spores of seasonal plants and fungi. In most parts of the United States, trees release their pollen in the spring, grasses in the late spring and summer, and weeds—particularly ragweed, perhaps the most notorious plant allergen of all—in the early fall. Mold spores are at their highest levels and, therefore, are the biggest problem for people with allergies when a rainy, damp, or foggy spell is followed by a warm, dry, windy period. These conditions can occur at any time, depending on where you live.

The seasonal pattern of pollen release and plant growth lets you predict when symptoms are likely to appear. This helps you plan when to take whatever preventive action your pediatrician may advise to lessen the impact.

HAY FEVER SYMPTOMS SHOULD NOT INCLUDE PAIN

Although at times hay fever symptoms seem to grip every part of the body in a feeling of general misery, they do not usually cause actual pain. If your child complains of pain in the face or mouth, a sensation of pressure, or headache, consult your pediatrician. The symptoms may indicate sinusitis, a dental problem, or another condition requiring treatment.

HAY FEVER: IT KEEPS GOING AND GOING AND GOING

Hay fever is not caused by seasonal allergens alone. Many people suffer year-round hay fever (your doctor calls it "perennial allergic rhinitis") because they are sensitive to allergens they encounter every day. Among the typical offenders are dust mites (see pp. 42,

76), indoor molds, and animal dander. It's hardly surprising that allergies are so common, because all three—mites, molds, and dander—are often present at high levels in many homes.

Although all the usual symptoms of hay fever may be present, for many children the most troubling symptom of year-round hay fever is a constantly stuffed-up nose. The child with year-round hay fever has difficulty breathing through the nose. Therefore, he takes the path of least resistance, breathing with an open mouth both day and night. These children may speak in an unmistakable nasal voice, and often have dry, cracked lips. They tend to eat noisily. They often snore at night, have broken sleep, and wake up in the morning with a dried-out, sore throat. They frequently cough to clear their throats throughout the day. Postnasal drip and cough are common complaints. The symptoms can become worse whenever a sensitive child is additionally exposed to seasonal plants and other allergens.

In the most common and uncomfortable pattern, the upper respiratory tract becomes chronically sensitized by allergens and remains so irritable that the least irritant—perhaps a draft of cool air, powdered ink from a photocopy, or a whiff of perfume—flings the child into spasms of sneezing. The nose becomes even more stuffed up and more drippy. What's more, in many areas, pollen and mold seasons last long enough to overlap, with the result that "seasonal" symptoms linger all year round.

WHEN A COLD ISN'T A COLD

It's sometimes difficult to know whether the problem is hay fever or a common cold (upper respiratory infection). The diagnosis is often made when parents seek their pediatrician's advice for a lingering "cold" that their child can't shake off. While symptoms of allergies and colds often overlap, there are a few telling differences. The tip-offs for hay fever are:
- A clear, watery nasal discharge.
- Itching of the eyes, ears, nose, and/or mouth.
- Spasmodic sneezing.

Fever is never part of the picture. If antibiotics are used, they don't help. Of course, antibiotics should not be used to treat a child with a cold; antibiotics are effective against bacteria, but not viruses, which cause colds. However, your pediatrician may prescribe an antibiotic if your child also has a bacterial infection, such as a sinus infection.

With a cold, unlike hay fever, the nasal secretions are thicker and somewhat colored. The child may have a sore throat and a cough, and the temperature is sometimes slightly raised, but not always. Itchiness is not usually a complaint with a cold, but it is the hallmark of an allergy problem.

SINUSITIS, EAR INFECTIONS, AND HAY FEVER

Year-round, or perennial, hay fever is closely linked to sinus infections and ear infections (otitis media) in children. Several factors are involved. Respiratory allergies cause congestion in the tissues, blocking the eustachian tubes (the tiny passages that run between the ear and the back of the throat) and the openings that allow secretions to drain from the sinus cavities. Persistent blockage of the eustachian tube causes an increase in secretions from the middle ear. Infected matter from the nose and throat can back up through the tube into the ear. Germs from this matter proliferate in the warm, moist environment, eventually causing an ear infection. Similarly, infections tend to develop in sinuses that are blocked and cannot drain.

Infants and young children are particularly susceptible because their eustachian tubes are not as functional as those in older children and adults. Children who are exposed to secondhand cigarette smoke are also vulnerable because substances in the smoke from tobacco not only irritate the lining of the respiratory tract and stimulate it to secrete protective mucus, but also interfere with the clearance of secretions.

Viral upper respiratory infections—in other words, colds—which are extremely common in young children, complicate the whole picture because they add further congestion and blockage.

Sometimes It's Fido, Sometimes Not

Furry pets are among the most common and potent causes of allergy symptoms. However, fur usually is not the only animal allergen. Even short-haired, "nonshedding" animals leave a trail of dander and saliva, as humans do. Cats are commonly more allergenic than dogs. Although certain breeds of dogs are said to be less allergenic than others, studies don't support this claim. Comparisons of dogs also show wide differences in allergenicity between individual dogs of the same breed. Reptiles, fish, and amphibians are not generally causes of allergy.

For families deeply attached to their animals, the notion of finding another home for a pet is hard to accept. Many prefer to keep the animal and battle on against allergy symptoms. If you can't part with your pet, at least keep it out of your allergic child's bedroom, and sweep, dust, and vacuum frequently. Another solution may be to keep your cat or dog permanently outdoors with adequate shelter. Weekly bathing in tepid water has also been shown to lower the allergenic potential of pets, including animals that never venture out of doors. Long after an animal has

With a sinus infection, congestion makes it difficult for the child to breathe through the nose and clear away the typical thick, discolored discharge. As a result, colds seem to promote bacterial ear and sinus infections more readily in children with allergies. The child with sinusitis often coughs at night, sleeps poorly, and consequently feels tired during the day. He may have bad breath. Sinusitis can also make asthma symptoms worse.

Quite often, chronic sinusitis—that is, a sinus infection that lasts for weeks— masquerades as year-round hay fever. As a result of long-standing infection, the nasal passages become persistently inflamed and irritable, with congestion similar to that seen in al-

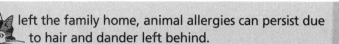

left the family home, animal allergies can persist due to hair and dander left behind.

It is unwise to adopt a furry pet if you have a strong family history of allergies and, consequently, a high risk that infants and young children in your home could develop allergies. Better to wait a few years and then, if there are no signs of trouble and skin tests are clear, look into pet adoption.

A household pet may be unjustly blamed for causing allergy symptoms. Don't automatically banish Fido to the doghouse unless the results of skin testing or RAST suggest that your child has an animal allergy.

Occasionally, symptoms that seem to be caused by an animal are, in fact, due to other allergies, such as dust mites or even plants. What happens is that Fido and Felix explore outdoors, then come back into the house with a load of pollens and spores in their coats. Every time the hay fever sufferer pats the pets, he stirs up an invisible cloud of allergens that triggers symptoms.

lergic rhinitis. There may be little or no discolored discharge if swelling has made the openings to the sinuses too narrow to allow mucus to drain, or if the mucus runs down the back of the throat. In an older child, some pain or tenderness may be felt in the face and around the teeth, but this is not always the case. As with hay fever, symptoms such as sneezing and runny nose occur all day long, and changes or irritants in the environment can make them worse. Only when a thorough workup for allergies proves negative and the doctor finds evidence of a sinus infection does a clear picture emerge. As the infection is treated, the "allergic" symptoms gradually resolve. In some cases, it's not only a question of allergies versus infection; both can be present at the same time. Antibiotics are prescribed to clear up bacterial ear infections and sinus infections. In some cases, your pediatrician may advise surgery, such as for removal of enlarged adenoid tissue or placement of tubes to allow ear drainage, or a procedure to drain the sinuses (also see p. 86). Often, when allergy-related inflammation inside the nose is properly controlled, an allergic child can avoid complications such as ear and sinus infections.

MANAGING HAY FEVER

As with other types of allergies, the ideal way to manage hay fever is to find out what your child is allergic to and then avoid it (for details about allergy testing see Chapter 2, "Establishing the Diagnosis," and about dealing with allergies, Chapter 7, "Approaches to Allergy Treatments"). It sounds simple, but this is much easier said than done. To start with, many children are allergic to pollens and molds, both of which are found everywhere outdoors and cannot be completely avoided. In addition, a child may be allergic to routinely encountered substances, such as dust mites or indoor molds. These everyday allergens can be kept at low levels when certain modifications are made. Still, they are almost impossible to eliminate altogether, no matter how meticulously you clean your home. Your child is also bound to run into allergens and irritants when he ventures out of your home and into other environments, such as school or friends' homes.

Exposure to plant allergens can be minimized by keeping your child indoors on days with high pollen and/or mold counts. It's helpful to use air conditioners, where possible, to reduce exposure to pollen in both your home and your car.

DUST MITES AND MOLDS. Dust had a reputation for causing sneezing and irritation long before allergies were called "allergies." Not only does it irritate the nose, throat, and eyes, but it can also contain allergenic materials. Recently, researchers have found that a major cause of allergic symptoms lies beyond the dust itself. It has been traced to dust mites—tiny creatures that, like Dr. Seuss's

"Roadblock Ahead!"

If your child has a runny nose with a discharge that:
- comes out of only one nostril,
- contains pus,
- smells bad,
- is tinged with blood,

there may be an object (a bead...a pea...a pebble...part of a toy) wedged inside the nose. Call your pediatrician and don't try to remove the object yourself.

Whos down in Whoville, make their homes among dust specks. But whereas the Whos asked only to be left in peace, there's no getting away from dust mites. They live wherever humans live and, in fact, they clean up after us. They can live on any organic debris, but their preferred diet is the half gram or so of worn-out skin cells that every human sheds daily. They also thrive on tiny fungi—like the mites, too small to be seen with the naked eye—that flourish where the relative humidity is fairly high, at 70 percent or more. Spores from these fungi are also a major cause of allergic symptoms in humans.

Dust mites congregate where food is plentiful. They are especially numerous in upholstered furniture, bedding, and rugs. Although vacuuming and dusting are important to keep irritants out of your home, these measures don't work very well against dust mites. Instead, a "containment" approach is needed. Choose blankets and pillows made of synthetic materials. Padded furnishings, such as mattresses, box springs, pillows, and cushions, should be encased in allergen-proof, zip-up covers, which are available through catalogs and specialized retailers (see Appendix 3, *Sources of Allergy and Asthma Products*, p. 175). Covers made of the newer, nonwoven synthetic fabrics are more comfortable than plastic covers and work at least as well. Since dust mites can survive in warm soapy water, wash linens weekly and other bedding, such as blankets, every 2 to 3 weeks in hot water. Then put them

Immunotherapy, or "allergy shots"—a series of injections of allergen extracts—can bring about substantial, long-lasting relief of hay fever by desensitizing children to the effects of allergen exposure. They work by giving small but increasing doses of the substances a person is allergic to, which gradually results in the person becoming less sensitive to the allergens.

The procedure can be time-consuming, but when successful it can reduce both symptoms and the need for medications. In some cases, it can prevent allergy episodes for an extended period. Immunotherapy is generally safe when carried out properly by experienced medical personnel. The most common side effects are swelling and redness at the site of the injection. More serious reactions, although rare, can occur, which is why allergy shots should be given in a medical office where reactions can be treated immediately. Allergy shots reduce allergen sensitivity in all parts of the body, so allergic reactions are suppressed in both the upper and lower respiratory tract and the eyes. As a bonus, the effects of treatment can persist long after treatment has been successfully completed.

Although many effective medications are now available to treat symptoms, some people prefer to try immunotherapy. The treatment is most cost-effective in those who are sensitive to airborne allergens, such as pollens. It is also more effective if steps are first taken to reduce exposure to environmental allergens, such as dust mites and animal dander, especially in the home.

through the hottest cycle of a clothes dryer. Pillows should be re-placed every 2 or 3 years.

Dust mites abound in cuddly stuffed toys. Where possible, replace soft, plush-covered toys with others that have smooth plastic bodies and washable clothes. If your child has a favorite soft toy that she can't be parted from, wash it every other day or so in hot water and dry it at the highest setting. Alternatively, seal soft toys in plastic bags and put them in the freezer for at least 5 hours or overnight once a week. Dust mites cannot survive longer than 5 hours at freezing temperature; you can then rinse the toys in warm water and put them in the dryer to get rid of the dead mites.

Keep bulky fabrics and dust-catching clutter out of your child's room. Remove wall-to-wall carpeting, if possible. Floors should be wooden or covered in another smooth material such as tile or vinyl. If you prefer rugs for comfort, use cotton or synthetic throw rugs that can be washed weekly in hot water. Curtains, too, should be easily washable. Chemicals designed to reduce levels of dust-mite allergens in carpet and upholstery (tannic acid-based sprays or acaricides) are available through catalogs and retailers of allergy products (see Appendix 3).

When it comes to the walls, the aim is to eliminate horizontal surfaces that trap dust. There should be no picture frames or shelves displaying books or ornaments, and all surfaces—on dressers, bedside tables, and other furniture—should be easy to wipe clean.

The use of a dehumidifier can help keep the humidity below the range that suits mites and molds. However, if you use a dehumidifier, it's essential not only to empty the water pan, but also to scour it daily to prevent the growth of invisible molds. High-efficiency particulate air (HEPA) cleaning devices are also useful for getting rid of airborne allergens. For a more detailed discussion, see Chapter 12, "How Environmental and Lifestyle Factors Affect Asthma."

No matter how careful you may be, you can't protect a child as if he were a hothouse plant. And even if you were to succeed in eliminating most environmental allergens, it's hard to avoid the normally harmless kinds of nonallergenic irritants that can set off symptoms in a nose already primed and "twitchy" due to allergen exposure.

MEDICATIONS. Long experience has shown that antihistamines are effective medications for relieving sneezing, itching, and runny nose due to seasonal hay fever (for details about medications used for allergy treatment, see Chapter 7). All antihistamines available without prescription have drowsiness as a possible side effect; your pediatrician may advise giving the dose at night so your child sleeps better and stays alert during school. Newer antihistamines, available only by prescription, are nonsedating. Antihistamines are less effective in year-round hay fever, especially where the major symptom is nasal congestion.

Decongestants are often prescribed together with antihistamines to unblock the nose in year-round hay fever. However, decongestants taken by mouth can have a number of side effects, making children feel overexcited and shaky or "jittery." These medications should be used very sparingly and only as prescribed by your pediatrician. Decongestants can be given as a nasal spray or nose drops, but if they are used too long, they can have a rebound effect, making the nose even more congested and irritated. This condition, called "rhinitis medicamentosa," is harder to treat than the original stuffy nose.

Corticosteroids given in the form of a nasal spray are the most effective medications currently available for reducing inflammation and congestion in the nose and relieving the symptoms of year-round hay fever. When used carefully, these medications often give better results than all other forms of medication treatment for allergic disease. Your pediatrician will prescribe the lowest possible dose to control the symptoms. He or she will closely monitor your child's progress to avoid side effects and may recommend periodic breaks in the treatment. (See Chapter 7 for details about treatments for allergy-related problems.)

CHAPTER 5

Food Allergies

At childcare, 2-year-old Justin is given a cracker with peanut butter by a fellow preschooler who wants to share. It is the first time Justin has ever eaten peanuts. Within 5 minutes of eating just a small amount, Justin develops mild wheezing. He also has swelling around his mouth and hives all over his body. The school administrator calls Justin's mother and by the time she arrives he is doing better. She immediately takes him to their pediatrician, who gives Justin an antihistamine medication for the hives and orders a RAST for peanuts, which comes back highly positive, confirming the suspicion that Justin is allergic to peanuts. The pediatrician advises that Justin must strictly avoid peanuts, and prescribes an epinephrine (adrenaline) autoinjection device for Justin's mother to

Food allergies are much less common than widely believed. Many of the symptoms that people believe to be food allergies are, in fact, problems of digestion or absorption. In contrast to allergies, these problems take place through mechanisms outside the immune system. Like allergies, however, they can often be managed simply by avoiding the food in question.

keep with her always, in case Justin ever accidentally swallows peanuts. Justin's mother also orders a bracelet for him to wear at all times, which identifies him as having severe peanut allergy. Everyone at the childcare center is alerted to make sure that Justin is never given peanuts to eat. His mother decides to eliminate peanut butter from their home when she learns that even a small amount left on a knife could end up contaminating Justin's food and causing a serious reaction. Life for Justin and his family will never be the same.

— ❖ —

Although many people use "food allergy"and "food intolerance" interchangeably, the terms describe two different conditions. Food allergy, also called food hypersensitivity, occurs because the immune system forms allergy antibodies to fight off a food, as if it were an alien threat. Each time the sensitized person eats the food, an antibody reaction leads to the release of histamine (see p. 4) and other chemicals that set off hives, itching, wheezing, and other allergy symptoms.

A food intolerance, by contrast, is a food-induced adverse reaction that does not involve the immune system. Lactose intolerance is a well-known example. People with lactose intolerance don't make enough lactase, an enzyme that is needed to digest lactose, the sugar in milk. When lactose-intolerant people drink milk or eat milk-based foods, they have symptoms affecting the digestive tract, such as gas, bloating, and stomachache.

Fortunately, many children outgrow food allergies. Whereas symptoms related to food affect up to 6 out of every 100 children at age 3, no more than 2 out of 100 are still having food allergy symptoms by age 10. However, food allergies that develop after age 3 are more likely to persist for life.

FOOD-ALLERGY SYMPTOMS

Symptoms of a food-allergy reaction can include vomiting, diarrhea, an itchy rash (ranging from just around the mouth and face to total-body hives), mouth and throat itchiness and swelling, difficulty breathing, and wheezing. Most true food-allergy reactions occur within minutes after ingesting the food.

The intensity of an allergic reaction may range from mild to severe at different times, partly depending on how much of an allergenic food your child eats. However, certain highly allergic children need to swallow only a very small amount of an offending food to be thrown into a violent allergic reaction. The way the food is prepared—whether processed or in its natural state, raw or cooked, hot or cold—can also affect the reaction. The severity of symptoms is influenced by the child's overall state of health, and whether she's exposed to just one allergen or several at the same time.

DIAGNOSING FOOD ALLERGIES

As with all forms of allergy, your pediatrician will review your child's medical history and question you closely about the foods he eats. Your pediatrician will also review your family's medical history for allergy-related conditions. He or she may order a RAST (see Chapter 2, "Establishing the Diagnosis") to identify specific food allergies, or send your child to a pediatric allergist for allergy skin testing. Both tests provide reliable information; however, one may be preferable to the other in some circumstances. For example, your physician will order a RAST rather than skin testing if eczema or other skin problems would make it difficult to read the results of skin tests.

Your pediatrician may also ask you to keep a food diary (see p. 21) for 2 to 4 weeks, noting every food your child eats, together with any symptoms that occur. If symptoms seem to be linked to a particular food, you may be advised to keep it out of your child's diet for a month to see if symptoms improve. There cannot be any slips at all in the diet during the trial period, or a trial of food elimination will not yield useful information. For example, if your pediatrician specifies "no eggs," that means no eggs in any form, including extracts in commercial food products (see "Eggs," p. 56, and Appendix 1, *Hidden Sources of Food Allergens*).

If the suspect food is an important source of nutrients such as vitamins or minerals, ask your pediatrician to recommend alternative sources.

Even though the results of skin tests and/or a RAST may help indicate one or more food sensitivities, positive skin test or RAST results do not always mean that your child is allergic to a food. Positive results must be interpreted by a professional experienced in diagnosing food allergy using all the available clinical information. Further, a skin test or a RAST may continue to give a positive result for a time after the child has outgrown that allergy.

MANAGING FOOD ALLERGIES

The appearance of food allergies can be delayed in some children who are at high risk because of a family history of allergies, if their mothers adhere to a systematic prevention plan. This plan starts from birth, with breastfeeding alone for at least the first 6 months and careful monitoring of the mother's diet to avoid foods known to cause allergies. The introduction of solid foods should be delayed somewhat longer than the 4 to 6 months the American Academy of Pediatrics recommends for nonallergic infants. When the child is weaned to solid foods, foods often associated with allergy are not introduced until the digestive and immune systems are mature enough to handle them. Although this approach may not prevent allergies, it appears to delay the appearance of allergy symptoms in some children.

Antihistamines and epinephrine (see Chapter 7, "Approaches to Allergy Treatments") can be used to treat symptoms after an allergenic food has been eaten by accident. However, allergy medications cannot be taken before a food is eaten to prevent symptoms. For now, allergy shots (immunotherapy, see p. 44) also cannot be used to prevent food allergy symptoms, but research is being done to develop preventive treatment.

If your pediatrician believes there is any risk that your child could have an anaphylactic reaction to food (anaphylaxis, see p. 6 and Chapter 6, "Killer Allergies: Anaphylaxis"), he or she will rec-

The Feingold Diet, Food Allergies, and ADHD

Years ago, the late Dr. Benjamin Feingold, a pediatric allergy specialist, theorized that the condition now known as attention deficit hyperactivity disorder (ADHD) was caused by certain food allergies. He developed a diet that he claimed would improve concentration and stop disruptive behavior in children diagnosed as having ADHD. The diet bans all foods that contain artificial colors and flavors (most commercially processed and packaged foods) as well as three widely used preservatives: BHA, BHT, and TBHQ. Also forbidden are foods that contain salicylates, the plant compounds on which aspirin is based. This category covers many fruits and vegetables, which are natural sources of salicylates.

Studies over more than two decades have shown that the Feingold diet does not control hyperactivity, although some parents insist that it helps their children. Specialists believe that if benefits occur, they do not come from the diet but, rather, from other factors, including the extra parental attention that children enjoy while on the diet.

In general, true food allergies do not appear to play a role in ADHD or other behavioral problems in children. However, if you are convinced that a particular food affects your child's behavior, note this and talk to your pediatrician to see whether he thinks it a good idea to pursue the question further.

ommend that you—and your child, when old enough to use it—always carry a preloaded epinephrine autoinjector ("beesting kit") in case of accidental contact with the allergen when outside your home or at school (see Appendix 1: *Hidden Sources of Food Allergens*). A child at risk for anaphylaxis should also wear a medical emergency identification tag at all times. For details about allergy treatment and prevention, see Chapter 7.

When children get out of hand, parents often blame sensitivity to candies and other high-sugar foods for the rambunctious behavior. Some even claim that sugar causes hyperactivity. However, the sugar-behavior link does not hold up to scientific scrutiny. The results of a carefully controlled study of preschool and school-age children showed no effect on behavior or concentration when the children's diet included far more sugar than normal, even among youngsters whose parents had identified them as "sugar sensitive." In another study, sugar had the opposite effect of what was predicted. When boys whose parents described them as "sugar reactive" were given large doses of sugar, they became less active than before. Studies comparing blood sugar (glucose) levels found that children with ADHD had exactly the same response to sugar as other children.

There is no scientific basis for the idea that sugar and other sweeteners cause ADHD or undesirable behavior. A moderate amount of sugar is acceptable in a balanced diet. But if your child acts oddly or has unusual symptoms after eating a particular food, it will do no harm to avoid it as long as his or her diet provides for choices from the same food group.

There's only one sure way to prevent food allergy symptoms, and that's by avoiding the problem food altogether, in all forms, at all times. A food that causes allergy may be one that your child has learned to avoid because he associates it with unpleasant symptoms. On the other hand, it may be a food that he really enjoys, despite the symptoms. In a long-term study of children who had vomiting because of a food allergy, some eventually outgrew the allergy and were able to eat the food without vomiting, and others avoided the food because it continued to cause vomiting, but one child enjoyed the food so much that he ate it even though it always made him vomit!

It's a fairly simple matter to keep a problem food away from a very young child, who eats meals and snacks under the watchful eye of parents or caregivers. However, it is more difficult with an older child, who has less supervision while eating. Not only your child but also his friends and their parents must be helped to understand how serious the condition is and how important it is to avoid the allergen in any form. Above all, children should be warned never to test whether claims of allergies are genuine by hiding a suspected allergen in another child's food.

Be sure to provide full information about the condition to school personnel and childcare providers. Update information regularly at the start of each school year and as new facts become available.

Because many children outgrow certain food allergies in their first 4 or 5 years, your pediatrician may suggest, at some point, that allergy testing be done on your child for the food that formerly caused problems. If the results are negative, a very small amount of the food may be given to your child in the doctor's office, where severe symptoms can be treated right away, should

THE FOOD ALLERGY NETWORK FOR UP-TO-DATE INFORMATION

The Food Allergy Network (FAN), a nonprofit organization, was established to increase awareness about food allergies and provide unbiased information and support for people with food allergies. The organization's main focus is on children, since food allergies are much more common in children than in adults. The FAN provides a variety of educational materials that may make it easier to approach your child's school.

Contact the FAN at www.foodallergy.org or (800) 929-4040. The address is: Food Allergy Network, 10400 Eaton Place, Suite 107, Fairfax, VA 22030-2208.

they occur. If your child doesn't develop symptoms, your physician may tell you it's safe to give small servings of the food at home. Then, if there are still no problems, he or she will tell you that your child may eat the food if he wants to. When the problem food is peanuts, tree nuts, or shellfish, testing and a food challenge may not be done, as these allergies tend to be lifelong and to cause the most serious reactions, including anaphylaxis.

BREASTFEEDING MAY HELP DELAY ALLERGY DEVELOPMENT

Breastfed babies tend to have fewer allergies, ear infections, and related problems than infants nourished on formula. That is one of the many reasons for which the American Academy of Pediatrics encourages mothers to breastfeed exclusively for the first 6 months (about the time your baby's diet begins to include solid foods) and to continue breastfeeding until at least 12 months or as long as baby and mother want to continue.

If there is a family history of asthma, eczema, hay fever, or other allergies, breastfeeding is especially important in reducing the risk of allergy development in an infant.

COMMON FOOD ALLERGENS

Any food may cause an allergic reaction, but 90 percent of food allergies in children are caused by just six foods: milk, eggs, peanuts, tree nuts, soy, and wheat. In adults, a similar percentage of allergies are caused by just four foods: peanuts, tree nuts, fish, and shellfish. Luckily, most children are allergic to only one food, which makes it easier to find a substitute when the allergenic food is an important source of nutrients (such as milk, a major source of calcium).

COW'S MILK. Allergy to cow's milk is among the most common hypersensitivities seen in young children, probably because it is the first foreign protein that many infants absorb, especially if they are bottle-fed. If cow's-milk allergy is present, occasionally even a breastfed infant may have colic or eczema until milk and dairy foods are eliminated from his mother's diet. Between 2 and 3 out of every 100 children younger than 3 years have allergy symptoms linked to cow's milk.

Vomiting after feeding is the most common way a child manifests milk allergy, but more severe reactions can occur. Colicky crying and gassiness can sometimes be the only indication of cow's-milk allergy in very young infants. (It must be said, though, that in the great majority of infants, no cause for colic is ever found, and the inconsolable crying eventually stops without treatment, never to return, before the baby is 6 months old.)[1] In addition, early symptoms often involve the typical itchy, dry rash of eczema (atopic dermatitis; see Chapter 3, "Skin Allergies"). Later, just as the eczema begins to fade, it's quite likely that the allergy will appear in a different form. Children with early milk allergy have a greater risk of developing respiratory allergies (hay fever, asthma) later on than those who are not allergic to milk as infants.

On learning that their child is allergic to cow's milk, some parents look to goat's milk, now widely available in supermarkets, as a substitute. However, at least half of all children who can't tolerate cow's milk are allergic to goat's milk. Even soy-based formula may be unsuitable for milk-allergic infants, because some who are sensitive to cow's milk are also unable to tolerate soy protein. If your milk-allergic child is a bottle-fed baby who still needs formula, your pediatrician will recommend a brand that is made with hydrolyzed protein, which is specially processed to be hypoallergenic.

Many children outgrow milk allergy as their immune systems mature, and milk and milk products often can be reintroduced

---

1 For more about colic and crying babies, see the American Academy of Pediatrics *Guide to Your Child's Symptoms,* Donald Schiff, M.D., and Steven P. Shelov, M.D., (editors), Villard Books, 1997, and *Guide to Your Child's Nutrition,* William H. Dietz, M.D., and Loraine Stern, M.D., (editors), Villard Books, 1998.

into the diet. However, your pediatrician will probably suggest that allergy tests be performed before your child tries milk again. Milk should first be given to your child in the doctor's office, where any reaction can be monitored and, if necessary, treated. If your child simply has lactose intolerance (see pp. 48 and 60), testing is usually unnecessary, and milk and milk products can be gradually reintroduced at home while you watch for reactions.

Milk and foods derived from milk are important sources of calcium, a mineral that's essential for strong bones and teeth, for muscle and nerve function, and for the health of every system in the body. Dark green leafy vegetables, canned fish eaten with the bones (sardines, salmon), calcium-fortified orange juice, dried figs and prunes, tofu, and dried beans are among the many rich nondairy sources of calcium for children who cannot tolerate milk, cheese, and yogurt.

EGGS. Pediatricians advise parents not to start children on whole eggs until after their first birthday to reduce the risk of allergy. Children who are allergic to eggs are reacting to the protein that's in the egg white but not in the yolk. However, because egg yolk can often be contaminated with egg white, it's safer for egg-allergic children to also avoid the yolk. Luckily, while eggs are nutritionally valuable and an excellent source of protein, they are not essential for good nutrition. Meat, fish, dairy products, and grains and legumes are also excellent sources of similar protein, minerals, and vitamins. If your child is allergic to eggs, he will have to avoid many commercially prepared foods, especially cakes, cookies, waffles, pancakes, French toast, and breads made with egg or glazed with egg wash.

Egg substitutes developed for low-cholesterol diets cannot be used. They are cholesterol-free but not totally egg-free, as they are made with egg white, the part responsible for causing allergies. Read food labels carefully to make sure ingredients do not include ovalbumin, ovamucin, or ovovitellin, all of which are egg-based products widely used in commercial food processing (also see Appendix 1 for additional sources of hidden food allergens).

PEANUTS AND TREE NUTS. When is a nut not a nut? When it's a legume—like peanuts, which are cousins to peas and beans. Like other legumes, peanuts grow on vines, not trees. Because peanuts and tree nuts come from different plant families, a child who is sensitive to peanuts can often eat walnuts, pecans, and other tree nuts without a problem. However, caution is needed because peanut-allergic children, for unknown reasons, are more likely also to have a separate tree-nut allergy.

When peanut allergy is present, it is often severe; a person with peanut allergy may have a serious reaction after merely kissing someone who has eaten peanuts or peanut butter. In this country, where people love peanuts and eat them in huge quantities, the most severe anaphylactic food reactions—fatal if not treated in time—occur in those who are allergic to peanuts and tree nuts.

Like eggs, peanuts are both delicious and nutritious, but they are not essential for a healthy diet. No nutritional substitutes are needed. Peanuts are often ground up and used as bulking agents in food products, such as candies. Read labels carefully to make sure that peanuts are not unsuspected ingredients in commercial foods. Occasionally, a label may note that the food has been packaged on equipment also used to package peanut-containing foods. Nut toppings for ice creams and baked goods are often made of deflavored peanuts that have been reflavored and colored to resemble more expensive tree nuts. If your child has a peanut allergy, avoid all chopped nuts to be safe. When eating out, be careful with fried foods. Although pure peanut oil, which is used for frying, is safe, traces of peanut protein—the allergenic component—may leach into the oil and cause trouble.

Allergy to tree nuts—walnuts, pecans, cashews, Brazil nuts, almonds, hazel nuts: all the nuts in hard shells—can be as severe as peanut allergy and the same warnings apply. Make caregivers, teachers, friends, and family members aware that your child must strictly avoid all products with even a trace of nuts and peanuts, including—for safety—salad dressings and baked goods made with unusual oils such as walnut, sesame, and grape seed, unless you are confident that they are 100 percent pure and safe.

If allergies run in your family, your pediatrician may recommend measures to prevent or delay the development of allergies in your infant.

- In most cases there's no need to restrict foods during pregnancy.

- Breastfeed exclusively for at least the first 6 months or use a low-allergenic formula (no cow's milk or soy protein), as your pediatrician advises.

- Introduce your baby to solid foods after 6 months of age, starting with rice cereal, nonleguminous (that is, not in the pea and bean family) vegetables, meats, noncitrus fruits and juices, preferably one at a time at monthly intervals.

- After age 1, add cow's milk, wheat, corn, citrus, and soy at monthly intervals.

- Wait until your child is at least 2 years old (some experts even say 3 years) before introducing peanuts (as smooth butter spread thin on bread or crackers; nuts, including chunky nut butters, should not be given to children younger than 4 because of the danger of choking), fish, and shellfish.

- If your child has symptoms indicating allergy after being given a particular food, keep it out of the diet and discuss the symptoms with your pediatrician.

SOY. A bottle-fed infant who develops a rash, runny nose, wheezing, diarrhea, or vomiting may be allergic to an ingredient of the formula, whether it is based on cow's milk (see p. 54) or soy. Colic—when the baby cries inconsolably, draws his knees up to the abdomen as if in pain, and passes gas—may also be related to allergy in some cases. Many infants who are allergic to cow's milk are also allergic to soy. Your pediatrician will recommend a low-allergenic, nonsoy, noncow's-milk formula made with hydrolyzed protein.

Ingredients derived from soybeans are widely used in commercially prepared foods. Read labels carefully. Be especially watchful for generic descriptions such as emulsifiers, stabilizers, lecithin, shortening, and vegetable oil; all of these may indicate that soy is the raw material. Of course, a child with soy allergy must avoid soy-based foods such as bean curd (tofu), miso soup and noodles, vegetable burgers and "hot dogs," and tempeh.

WHEAT AND GLUTEN. Rice and oats are usually the first cereals introduced into the diet, as they are less likely than other grains to cause allergy problems. If there are no problems with oats, wheat is given next. Wheat is the grain that is most often associated with allergies, but even so, it is an uncommon food allergy. This is fortunate because wheat is found in so many prepared foods.

There are two types of wheat allergy. In the first, food allergy symptoms such as hives or wheezing occur immediately after the child eats a food made with wheat.

The second type of wheat allergy is called celiac sprue, gluten intolerance, or gluten-sensitive enteropathy. Gluten is a protein found in wheat, rye, and, to a lesser extent, oats and barley. In a sensitive child, gluten damages the lining of the small intestine and interferes with the absorption of nutrients. Typical symptoms of celiac sprue are abdominal pain, diarrhea, irritability, and slow growth or even weight loss. Gluten intolerance may be diagnosed shortly after the infant has his first bowl of cereal, but in some cases, the symptoms are so minor that the conditions can smolder at a low level for years and a diagnosis may not be made until adolescence or even adulthood. Fortunately, the condition is rare.

CORN. Corn allergy is rarely encountered. If skin tests or a RAST suggest corn allergy in your child, read food labels carefully. Corn-based ingredients are widely used in commercial foods, snacks, and soft drinks. Corn is popular, but not a rich source of nutrients. You do not need to make up for the lack of it in your child's diet.

LACTOSE INTOLERANCE

Lactose intolerance is not an allergy. It's a digestive problem—an inability to digest lactose, the sugar in milk. People with lactose intolerance have low levels of an enzyme, lactase, which is normally produced in the lining of the small intestine. When there is not enough lactase to break down lactose into forms that can be easily absorbed, the milk sugar ferments in the intestine, causing cramps, bloating, gas (flatulence), diarrhea, and nausea anywhere from about 30 minutes to 2 hours after a meal. The symptoms of lactose intolerance are never serious or life-threatening, but they can be uncomfortable.

If your pediatrician suspects lactose intolerance as the cause of symptoms, your child may be referred for diagnostic tests. However, it's a straightforward matter to diagnose lactose intolerance. Your pediatrician may simply suggest that you reduce milk and milk foods or eliminate them entirely for 2 to 4 weeks. If your child's symptoms go away, the diagnosis is established.

Lactose intolerance is not unusual. In fact, it gradually develops in most of the world's population after about 3 or 4 years of age, when milk is no longer a major part of the diet. However, the condition is fairly unusual in those whose ancestors came from Northern Europe. It's rare for a baby to be born with lactose intolerance, but a toddler or older child may have trouble digesting milk for a week or two after a bout of diarrhea or following treatment with an antibiotic, both of which can temporarily affect the ability to produce lactase.

Symptoms of lactose intolerance are fairly easy to manage with dietary measures. Most supermarkets sell lactose-reduced milk and other dairy foods. The milk retains all the ingredients of regular milk and can be kept the same length of time in the refrigerator. Lactase enzyme tablets or liquid can be added to milk at home to reduce the lactose content by about 70 percent. Chewable tablets taken before a meal are available to help digest solid foods that contain lactose.

A young child with lactose intolerance should avoid foods containing lactose, including milk, yogurt, ice cream, and cheese. If milk is ruled out altogether, your pediatrician will suggest alternative sources for calcium, as for children with cow's-milk allergy. Older children can usually eat small amounts of lactose-containing foods, particularly if the foods are part of a meal and not eaten alone. Many children can enjoy aged cheeses and yogurts, where the lactose is naturally broken down in the manufacturing process. As time goes on, your child will be able to gauge, by trial and error, the amount of milk or milk-based foods she can handle.

CHAPTER 6

Killer Allergies:
Anaphylaxis

T en-year-old Bryan likes to play around the ice plant in his backyard, a spot that also attracts many bees. Once, when running barefoot, Bryan is stung on his foot by a bee. Soon afterward he develops mild hives over most of his body, and has some swelling in the area of the sting. His mother calls their pediatrician, who tells her to give the youngster an antihistamine and come to the office. Bryan responds so well—the hives quickly go away—that she decides not to bother to go in.

Next time, Bryan is stung on the hand. Immediately, he goes into the house to find his mother. His chest feels tight, he is wheezing, and his throat feels swollen and itchy. His mother immediately takes him to the nearest hospital emergency department, where he is treated with epinephrine (adrenaline) and given antihistamine intravenously so the medication can be quickly absorbed.

When Bryan's symptoms are under control, the emergency medicine physician explains that the attack was a severe form of

> *A*naphylaxis is the most intense form of allergic reaction, but luckily, also the rarest. It comes on without warning, causes severe symptoms, and may lead to death unless treated. Anaphylaxis is always an emergency and requires immediate medical attention.

allergy known as "anaphylaxis." She prescribes preloaded epinephrine autoinjectors: a couple for Bryan's mother to keep in the house and the car, and another for Bryan to carry with him at all times in case he is stung again.

At a follow-up appointment, their pediatrician refers Bryan for evaluation by an allergy specialist. The results of allergy skin testing shows that Bryan is highly allergic to honeybee venom. The allergy specialist makes sure that Bryan and his parents all know exactly how and when to use the epinephrine autoinjector. The doctor also recommends that Bryan start allergy shots (immunotherapy) to desensitize him to bee venom.

— ❖ —

Anaphylaxis, like less severe forms of allergy, is a rare overreaction by the immune system to invasion by a foreign allergen. But while less severe allergies may affect one or more body systems and occur more or less gradually, such as when a child has eczema on the skin and/or wheezing in the airways, anaphylaxis can take over every system at once with sudden, full-force symptoms.

Within minutes of being exposed to an allergen, a youngster in the throes of anaphylaxis may turn bright red, break out in hives, have marked swelling (angioedema, see p. 32) of the face, especially the lips and eyes, and inside the mouth, throat, and voice box. The reaction causes the smooth muscles of the lungs—these are involuntary muscles—to go into spasm, closing down the air-

EMERGENCY HELP FOR ANAPHYLAXIS

If you suspect your child is having anaphylaxis (he's suddenly weak, pale, and short of breath, and has a rash or widespread swelling), call the Emergency Medical Service (911 in most areas) immediately. If your child stops breathing or you can't feel a pulse, start cardiopulmonary resuscitation (CPR) as soon as you have called for help.

Many substances have the potential to cause anaphylaxis, but it can't be stressed enough that anaphylaxis is rare. The chances of your child having an anaphylactic reaction are quite remote. However, this severe type of allergic reaction is something everyone should be able to recognize, in order to know when to get emergency help, whether for your own child or somebody else's.

ways. The child wheezes as she gasps for breath. Her blood pressure drops, her pulse races, and her skin turns clammy. She may be overcome by nausea, vomiting, and diarrhea. In severe anaphylaxis, the child goes into shock, her blood vessels relax, preventing the heart from maintaining normal blood pressure.

An identical type of sudden, rare reaction can occur that does not involve the IgE allergy antibodies (see p. 4). This is called an "anaphylactoid" reaction, which means that it is like anaphylaxis, though caused by a different mechanism. It may come on during exercise, or when a susceptible youngster takes certain medications, such as aspirin or another nonsteroidal anti-inflammatory drug (NSAID). The symptoms are the same as those of anaphylaxis and an attack requires the same prompt emergency measures.

Researchers believe that, in general, the sooner symptoms appear, the more severe an attack of anaphylaxis is likely to be. In some cases, an attack occurs in two phases. Treatment is given and the symptoms clear up, only to reappear with the same intensity after a lapse of several hours. The physician treating a child for anaphylaxis will keep her under observation or warn caregivers to watch her carefully until the danger period has passed.

RISK FACTORS FOR ANAPHYLAXIS

Unless a youngster has previously had a warning episode with severe allergic symptoms, it's impossible to foresee when anaphylaxis may strike. However, there are certain conditions that—even if they don't actually cause anaphylaxis—tend to be found more often in those who experience attacks. They are warning signals to watch for.

ALLERGIES. Although anaphylaxis or an anaphylactoid reaction can occur in a person with no previously identified allergies (such as to penicillin or beestings), generally, people who experience anaphylaxis are more likely to have a history of allergies than the general population.

LIFESAVING TECHNIQUES

Even though rescue breathing is not used in asthma and allergy treatment, every parent and caregiver should know how to do three critical lifesaving techniques: cardiopulmonary resuscitation (CPR), the infant CPR/choking procedure, and the Heimlich maneuver for choking in older children. Local chapters of the American Red Cross and the American Heart Association, many hospitals and medical centers, and local fire departments offer courses on these techniques. Video stores rent out cassettes for refresher courses.

TYPE OF ALLERGEN. Again, for undetermined reasons, certain allergens are more often involved in anaphylaxis. Food (for example peanuts, milk, eggs, tree nuts) and insect venom (especially bee) are the leading causes of anaphylactic reactions among children. Much less common causes are antibiotics (such as penicillin) and latex. These same allergens plus shellfish are frequent causes in adults; shellfish causes fewer problems in children, possibly because children eat shellfish less often.

When a youngster is allergic to medication—commonly, an antibiotic in the penicillin family—the risk of anaphylaxis is higher if the dose is given by injection, rather than by mouth.

FREQUENCY OF CONTACT. The risk of anaphylaxis seems to be higher when a youngster has had several brief exposures to an allergenic substance, followed by a long contact-free lull. The next contact, after this interval, is the one that may trip the wire for an anaphylactic episode. Also, the more often a person comes in contact with a potentially allergenic substance, the higher the statistical chances that an anaphylactic reaction could occur. But, as noted earlier, anaphylaxis is highly unpredictable, and an attack may occur in the rare child who has no previous known contact with the allergen.

Side Effects of Medications Are Not Allergy Symptoms

Mild stomach upset is sometimes a side effect of antibiotic treatment, but it is not an allergic reaction. If you have difficulty telling normal side effects from allergy symptoms, ask your pediatrician to explain the difference. If your child has any unusual reaction, after taking medication, call your pediatrician at once.

Where Does Anaphylaxis Come From?

Although almost any substance could cause anaphylaxis, those that most often do so fall into just four categories. The leading anaphylaxis triggers in children have been narrowed down to the following four categories:

- Foods.
- Insect stings and bites.
- Medications.
- Latex.

Rare as anaphylaxis is to begin with, other known causes, such as exercise, are especially rare in adults and almost unheard of in children. In some cases, a cause is never identified. This type of reaction is called "idiopathic anaphylaxis."

Keep Your Child's School Informed About Anaphylaxis

Let teachers and school personnel know if your child is severely allergic and is at risk for anaphylaxis. Make sure teachers know what symptoms to look for and what measures to take. Give your child an epinephrine (adrenaline) autoinjector to carry at all times, and talk to the school nurse to make sure she is familiar with emergency measures.

Foods

Peanuts, milk, eggs, and tree nuts are the most common food triggers for childhood allergy (see Chapter 5, "Food Allergies") and anaphylaxis. Peanuts are a leading cause of anaphylaxis in all age groups in the United States, and peanut allergy, unlike egg and milk allergies, is rarely outgrown. Because peanuts are legumes, related to peas and beans but not to tree nuts, a child who is allergic to peanuts is not necessarily allergic to tree nuts and may be able to eat them. However, there is a danger that peanuts may sometimes be "snuck in" with tree nuts. Parents and children who are allergic to peanuts and/or tree nuts need to read food labels carefully and be aware that nuts are hidden ingredients in many foods (see p. 57 and Appendix 1, *Hidden Sources of Food Allergens*).

Milk and foods containing milk protein are often the cause of anaphylaxis among babies and toddlers, because milk is such an important part of their diet. Although egg white is the main allergy and anaphylaxis trigger in egg-allergic children, a youngster who is highly allergic should avoid yolks as well, since the yolk may be contaminated by traces of protein from the white.

Sometimes it's difficult to know which food set off a severe reaction. Your pediatrician may use a RAST or refer your child for skin tests (see Chapter 2, "Establishing the Diagnosis") to identify your child's food allergies.

INSECT STINGS AND BITES

The risk of insect stings has been known, if not understood, for a very long time. Almost 5,000 years ago, scribes recorded the death of an Egyptian king who collapsed after a wasp or hornet sting. Insect stings—which are injections, like some medications—cause pain and swelling whether your child is allergic or not. An allergic child may break out in hives or have unusual swelling, but the risk of anaphylaxis because of insect-venom allergy is quite small.

Honeybees are the main offenders; hornets, yellow jackets, and wasps can also deliver a potentially lethal venom. Fire ants are a growing problem, especially in the South and Southwest. Deer flies and some other biting insects have also rarely been linked to anaphylaxis. However, although bites from houseflies, mosquitoes, fleas, and ticks can cause symptoms ranging from a mild, itchy nuisance to Lyme disease (a potentially serious disorder caused by germs carried by deer ticks), they never lead to life-threatening allergic reactions.

WHEN TO GET HELP. Your child may have severe pain and swelling after an insect sting, but there is no cause for alarm as long as the reaction stays localized to the site of the sting. Hives that occur immediately after an insect sting warrant seeking medical help, but as long as there are no other serious symptoms, such as breathing difficulties, the child usually does just fine. However, if your child has the typical skin symptoms plus symptoms in another part of the body (such as wheezing, hoarseness, or a swelling sensation inside the mouth or throat), call 911 (the Emergency Medical Service, EMS) at once. The results of anaphylaxis are so serious that, when in doubt, doctors always treat rather than wait and see.

Even if anaphylaxis does not develop, report severe or unusual symptoms to your pediatrician, who may refer your child to a pediatric allergy specialist to perform allergy tests to identify or confirm your child's sensitivity.

If your doctor believes there is a risk of anaphylaxis, he or she will prescribe an epinephrine (adrenaline) autoinjector for you (and your child when he or she is old enough to use it) to carry at all times and will tell you how to use it in emergencies. Your child should wear a medical identification tag specifying what she is allergic to.

ALLERGY SHOTS FOR INSECT STINGS. If the results of tests show that your child has an insect-sting allergy, your pediatrician may recommend allergy shots (venom immunotherapy), which give good protection against future reactions.

Venom immunotherapy enables the insect-allergic child to develop immunity to the insect venom, preventing the venom from

Protect Your Child from Insect Stings

- For outside play, dress your insect-allergic child, when you can, in a long-sleeved shirt, long pants, and shoes and socks. A broad-brimmed hat can help to keep insects away from the face.

- Avoid bright-colored clothes, perfume, or aftershave lotion, which can attract insects.

- Apply insect repellent to your child's clothing, not the skin. Read the label to check that repellent contains no more than 10 percent DEET. DEET is effective but can be harmful when absorbed through the skin.

- Oils of citronella and peppermint are natural insect repellents that can be mixed with vegetable oil and applied to clothing.

- Keep door and window screens in good repair.

- Warn your child when outside to avoid areas that attract flying insects, such as beds of flowers and succulents such as ice plant, flowering shrubs, fruit trees and bushes, and garbage containers.

- When eating outside, such as at picnics, check fruits and sweet foods for insects. Look inside cans and bottles before drinking.

setting off the child's allergic mechanisms. This reduces the risk that the child will have a serious allergic reaction after future insect stings.

The treatment is given by injecting gradually stronger doses of insect venom into the child's arm over an extended period. Injections are given once or twice a week at first, then at longer intervals. When the venom strength has reached a predetermined goal, the child gets a "maintenance" injection once a month to keep up a good level of protection (also see Chapter 7, "Approaches to Allergy Treatments").

BEE-STING AND PENICILLIN ALLERGIES DON'T SEEM TO RUN IN FAMILIES

Although a tendency of allergies runs in many families, family history and genetics do not seem to be important in penicillin and bee-sting allergies. In other words, although either parent may have had a severe allergic reaction to a bee sting or to treatment with amoxicillin (an antibiotic related to penicillin), their child does not have an increased risk of having a bad reaction. The tendency does not run in families.

MEDICATIONS

Many different medications have been linked to anaphylaxis attacks. It's not surprising that penicillin and some related antibiotics are often implicated, because bacterial infections requiring antibiotic treatment are among the most frequent childhood illnesses. Some children who are allergic to penicillin may also have an allergic cross-reaction when given one of a related group of antibiotics, the cephalosporins, although such cross-reactions are rare. Anaphylaxis can occur no matter how a medication is given, but happens more often after injections.

Unless your child has a proven sensitivity to penicillin or an-

What to Do If You Suspect Your Child Is Having an Anaphylactic Reaction After an Insect Sting

- Try to stay calm.
- Call or have someone else call 911 (Emergency Medical Service).
- Use your epinephrine (adrenaline) injector, if one has been prescribed.
- Give an antihistamine if you have one available.
- Go at once to where there are other people.
- Wait for the EMS or take the child immediately to the nearest emergency department.
- If your child stops breathing, or you can't feel your child's pulse, start CPR at once while you wait for the EMS.

other medication, there is little need to worry about the possibility of a reaction. Most medications are safe, and a serious reaction is unlikely to happen more than once in several million doses.

Your pediatrician keeps a record of your child's allergies on file but, in any case, will always ask about medication allergies before writing a prescription. There are usually several effective alternatives for any medication that your child cannot take because of allergy symptoms.

LATEX

The numbers of people allergic to latex are rising, as latex gloves are increasingly used to protect against the spread of infections. Some allergens occur naturally in raw latex, while others are by-products of the manufacturing processes that turn the gummy sap into useful products. There are two types of latex allergy. The more common type is contact, also called "delayed-type allergy," which comes on gradually and usually causes skin symptoms on the hands. It is a nuisance but not a disabling problem. The second, termed "immediate-type allergy," is more serious and can result in anaphylaxis.

Symptoms of immediate-type allergy may occur when an allergic person touches latex, breathes in tiny particles, or is exposed to latex during surgery, dental work, or contact with other medical personnel who use latex gloves. Be sure to warn your child's dentist if your child has been diagnosed as having immediate-type latex allergy.

Those with latex allergy have an increased risk of allergies to several foods. They should be careful with bananas, kiwi fruit, chestnuts, and avocados, as allergic reactions—including anaphylaxis—to these foods have occurred in latex-sensitive people.

CHAPTER 7

Approaches to Allergy Treatments

Marissa and her parents are thrilled at the improvement in the teenager's overall well-being. About nine months ago, the family pediatrician referred Marissa to an allergy specialist who diagnosed her as having chronic allergic rhinitis, or "hay fever." Many people have hay fever in the spring and summer, when pollen is heavy, but Marissa has the typical symptoms of runny, itchy nose, itchy eyes, and sneezing all year round. In addition, her hay fever symptoms were worsened by frequent sinus infections. The results of skin tests and a RAST confirmed that the teenager was allergic to many substances found both outdoors and indoors, including dust mites, cat dander, mold, and grass pollen.

The allergy specialist put Marissa on a three-prong treatment plan. He recommended several measures to control dust in her bedroom, advised against using a humidifier in the house, and asked that

In the best-case scenario, the ideal treatment for allergies is to avoid the substances that trigger symptoms. Of course, this is often impossible because many allergens are always in the air around us. Fortunately we now have an array of effective medications that help control symptoms. And if medications don't do the trick, allergy shots (immunotherapy) are another solution.

the family cat be kept entirely outdoors. In addition, the physician instructed Marissa to use a cortisone nasal spray and take an antihistamine tablet every morning. He also prescribed a decongestant nasal spray for Marissa to use only when she felt sinus congestion or an infection developing. In the hope of being able to control her allergies with fewer medications over time, Marissa decided to start immunotherapy (allergy shots) and has faithfully kept to the schedule for eight months.

Now everything seems to be falling into place: Marissa's nose symptoms are much less severe, she doesn't need to stay near a tissue box, she is sleeping better, and she feels that she has more energy. What's more, Marissa hasn't had a single sinus infection since starting the treatment program.

Physicians employ a three-point strategy to control allergies:
1. Avoidance to reduce allergen exposure.
2. Medications to control and prevent symptoms.
3. Allergen-specific immunotherapy (allergy shots), where appropriate, to decrease children's sensitivity.

ALLERGEN AVOIDANCE TO REDUCE EXPOSURE

Allergen avoidance begins at home for two important reasons. First, home is where it's easiest to control conditions. And second, indoor allergens found in our homes (see box on p. 75, *Common Allergens on the Home Front*) are often the main causes of symptoms. That's because they are often present at fairly high levels even when a home is regularly cleaned. Moreover, children are exposed to them repeatedly and for long periods because home is where children spend most of their time. Measures to reduce allergen exposure may take some planning and effort, but they can often be achieved at little or no expense and offer a cost-effective way to prevent allergy symptoms.

DUST CONTROL. When you know that dust is among the causes of your child's allergic symptoms, you may want to reach for the vacuum cleaner every time you spy a trace of dust on the furniture. But vacuuming may not be the solution. Use of a normally effi-

COMMON ALLERGENS ON THE HOME FRONT

- Dust (contains dust mites and finely ground particles from other allergens such as cockroaches, pollen, mold, and animal dander)
- Pollen (trees, grasses, weeds)
- Fungi (including molds too small to be seen with the naked eye)
- Furry animals (cats, dogs, guinea pigs, gerbils, rabbits, and other pets)
- Clothing and toys made, trimmed, or stuffed with animal hair
- Latex (household articles such as rubber gloves, toys, balloons; elastic in socks, underwear, and other clothing; airborne particles)
- Seed dusts (beanbag toys and cushions)
- Bacterial enzymes (used to manufacture enzyme bleaches and cleaning products)
- Foods
- Airborne dust from grain elevators, barns, and haylofts (in rural areas)

cient vacuum cleaner stirs up clouds of fine dust that can hang about in the air for up to eight hours and make sneezing, runny nose, and itchiness worse. It's best to wait until your allergic child is out of the house—at school for the day, for example—before vacuuming. Or, to avoid stirring up dust, invest in a vacuum cleaner with a high-efficiency particulate air (HEPA) filter. To keep household dust levels down, clean all noncarpeted floors at least once a week with a damp mop and use a damp cloth to wipe flat surfaces, louver blinds, window ledges, and picture frames.

Air-conditioning is the most efficient way to keep your home free of allergens and irritants brought in by air from the outside. While it may be too costly to install air-conditioning throughout your home, you may find an economical way to install a unit in your allergic child's bedroom. This could help him sleep better at

Dust mites are felt to be the main source of allergens in house dust. It's difficult for many people who are allergic to accept that these creatures, invisible except under a microscope, can be present in large numbers even in a thoroughly cleaned home. Some are convinced only when symptoms improve as a result of drastic mite-containment measures.

Dust mites are members of the same family as spiders. Too small to be seen with the naked eye, they find a home wherever humans live. Dust mites don't ask for much in life. They feed on any protein that comes their way, and find easy pickings in the dead skin scales that humans shed every day. Apart from this simple diet, they need only a moderately warm, moist atmosphere, with a temperature of 65°F or higher, and humidity around 65 percent. Bedding is the ideal dust-mite home; after all, bedding offers warmth, sufficient moisture, plenty of skin, and fibrous materials to which dust mites can cling with their barbed legs. They also thrive in upholstered furniture, clothing, soft toys, and carpets.

The dust mite eats, excretes pellets of feces that are about the size of pollen grains, and finds other dust mites, with which it produces many offspring. Their fecal pellets enter the general household dust to become the main source of allergens. Eventually, as mites die off, their dried-out carcasses, composed of allergenic proteins, also join the dust.

night and provide a low-allergen retreat on days when the pollen count is high. Air-conditioner filters should be checked and cleaned regularly, and sprayed with an antimildew aerosol to control the growth of molds.

Families may find that their allergic members have fewer symptoms when room air is filtered through a HEPA air cleaner. However, air filtration should complement, not replace, measures to control mites. A HEPA air cleaner can be installed centrally in a forced-air ventilation system, or used as a portable room unit and left on at night in your child's bedroom (also see next section). When you run a room HEPA cleaning unit, make sure that the windows of the room are shut and the bedroom door is closed.

YOUR ALLERGIC CHILD'S BEDROOM. Since your allergic child spends more time in the bedroom than in any other single location, it's a good idea to begin allergen control there. But if your child is highly allergic or several members of the family suffer from allergy symptoms, you may decide to extend many of the suggestions for allergen control from the bedroom throughout the rest of the house. Modifications suggested for the bedroom generally apply to other rooms as well.

The watchword for allergen control should be "Simplify!" Throughout your home, get rid of dust catchers and put out-of-season clothing and articles that are used only occasionally into accessible storage. Use bedroom storage only for clothing and objects in current use.

Canopy beds and bunk beds are not good choices for allergic youngsters. The drapes on canopy beds are dust catchers, and bunk beds release an invisible shower of dust and mites over the lower bunk every time the child in the top bunk stirs in his sleep.

All beds in the bedroom should be treated identically, including spare beds that are only occasionally used. Mattresses, box springs, and pillows should be encased in vinyl-backed, dustproof zippered casings. Seal zippers all along their length with duct tape to prevent leakage of dust mites and other allergens. Vinyl-backed casings for bedding are available through catalogs, specialized retailers, and bedding departments of some major retailers (see Appendix 3, *Sources of Allergy and Asthma Products*). A waterbed may be better than a regular bed for a child who is allergic to dust mites. However, some waterbeds are unsuitable because they have quilting or padding that can harbor dust mites. Vacuuming is not an efficient way to remove live mites from carpeting and bedding. However, once dead, the mites cling less to their fibrous homes and are somewhat easier to vacuum up.

Benzyl benzoate foam or powder and other allergy products obtainable through catalogs and specialized retailers, applied periodically, will also lower levels of mite allergens in carpets and upholstered furniture. Follow the safety directions on containers to reduce your family's exposure to the chemicals. Benzyl benzoate, for example, should not be inhaled by anyone of any age, nor should it come in contact with the skin. To be safe, children should not be in the house while it is being applied and until after it is vacuumed up.

KEEP HUMIDITY LOW TO DISCOURAGE MITES

Dust mites flourish when the humidity is around 75 to 80 percent. These tiny cousins of spiders need water to survive but have no means of conserving it in their tissues. When the surrounding humidity falls below 50 percent, the mites soon shrivel up and die. Thus, reducing household humidity can drastically reduce the dust-mite population. A dehumidifier is useful for drying out the air. Take care to empty the water pan daily and scour it to stop the growth of microscopic molds (also see p. 76).

Avoid pillows, comforters, and cushions stuffed with down, feathers, or kapok. Replace woolen blankets with washable synthetics. Use only pillows and comforters stuffed with man-made fibers and replace pillows every 2 to 3 years. Your child should take his own pillow on sleepovers and when traveling.

Use only synthetic or easily washable, lightweight, natural-fiber fabrics to furnish your child's room. Mites and molds multiply in natural materials such as wool and wicker. Fabrics should be flat-weave (like percale and chintz), not napped (like chenille

USE OF A HUMIDIFIER CAN PROMOTE GROWTH OF MITES AND MOLDS

Any increase in humidity, such as when a humidifier is used, will encourage mites and molds to grow in your child's room. If your child has problems with croup or other breathing difficulties, ask your pediatrician's advice about the best way to ensure that the air in the bedroom is moist enough to breathe comfortably, but dry enough to discourage mites and molds.

and velour). Sheets and pillowcases should, of course, be washed weekly, and all other bedding every 2 or 3 weeks. Dust mites can survive a lengthy wash in warm, soapy water. Wash all bedding for no less than 10 minutes in hot water, then place it in the dryer at the highest setting to kill any remaining dust mites. Although many people prefer the feel and smell of laundry fresh from the clothesline, laundry dried outdoors can worsen allergies, because pollens and other airborne allergens collect on the clothes and bedding.

Check your child's toy box periodically and get rid of toys that are no longer wanted or being used. Sweep the toy box and air it out from time to time to get rid of dust and prevent mold growth. Wash plastic toys periodically in soapy water or put them through a cycle in the dishwasher, if you have one. If your child can't be parted from a favorite soft toy, wash it regularly in hot water with the bedding, or seal it in a plastic bag and leave it in the freezer overnight once a week to kill dust mites (also see p. 76).

Unframed maps, posters, and prints can be used to brighten up the walls, but fabric pennants and hangings, three-dimensional sculptural decorations, and picture frames catch dust and are best kept for another part of the house or relegated to storage. Sadly, books harbor molds, and bookshelves gather dust. Store books in another room (dust them regularly) and try to keep only the current issues of newspapers, magazines, and comics.

Houseplants should be kept out of your child's room. Some allergy specialists advise getting rid of potted plants in all areas of the house, although others disagree that plants are a major source of molds. If you cultivate houseplants, rinse the leaves regularly, both for the plants' sake and to keep dust away from your allergic child.

Mildew-resistant paint is a better choice for bedroom walls than wallpaper. Molds can grow on the paper and in the adhesive paste.

To keep out pollen and environmental contaminants, your child's bedroom windows should be left closed as much as possible. Lightweight, washable curtains and/or vertical vinyl shades are suitable window coverings. Curtains should be washed at least once a month and vinyl shades dusted weekly with a damp sponge or dust-retentive tack cloth. Shutters, venetian and other "horizontal" blinds, drapes, and elaborate valances are not the best choice for your allergic child's bedroom; they are dust traps that may make allergy symptoms worse.

Bare wood, tile, and vinyl or linoleum are best for bedroom floors. Choose flat-weave or low-pile area and accent rugs made of cotton or synthetic fiber in small sizes that make it easy to wash and dry them frequently.

Avoid using potpourri, incense, and solid, wick, or spray room deodorizers. Potpourri can harbor molds and may contain spices and other irritating or allergenic particles that enter the air. The smell from room deodorizers can irritate sensitive mucous membranes in the nose of an allergic child or irritate the airways of a child with asthma.

HEATING SYSTEMS. Dust and molds collect in heating ducts and fill the air when the furnace is in operation. Baseboard heating and radiant heat are preferable to forced-air systems in homes where people have allergies. Unfortunately, the cost of replacing a heating system is more than most families can manage. Where possible, the best solution is to seal off the heating vents in your child's bedroom with aluminum covers and tape to prevent dust-laden air from entering. The air ducts to the rest of the house should be cleaned regularly. Ask your heating company to replace the standard fiberglass furnace filters with more efficient filters that are better traps for dust and allergens.

ANIMAL ALLERGIES. Cats and dogs are among the most frequent causes of allergies (also see p. 75). If your child is sensitive to other allergens, there is a good chance that with a pet—especially an indoor pet—in the home, she will also develop an animal allergy sooner or later.

When the family history makes it likely that a baby or young child will develop allergies, it's best to postpone adopting a pet for several years until you are certain that your child is not allergic. In the case of an animal that has been part of the family since before the arrival of a child with allergies, decisions can be more difficult, especially when older children have formed strong attachments to the pet.

Where allergies are severe, the kindest course is to find a new home for the animal. However, if you can't part with your pet, provide shelter and restraints to let it live outside. If this is not a practical solution, groom and bathe the animal frequently to reduce shedding of allergenic particles and hair, and keep it strictly out of your allergic child's bedroom and play areas. When considering a pet, look into the possibility of an unusual but easily maintained animal. For example, allergic children rarely have problems with fish or with reptiles in a terrarium.

Give teachers and school personnel full information about your child's animal allergies. A highly allergic child may develop symptoms if animals (typically, rabbits, birds, or small rodents) live in the classroom or come to school on visits. Made aware of the severity of your child's symptoms, teachers may reconsider the type of classroom animal (perhaps turtles or lizards instead of gerbils) and make sure that animals brought on special visits stay in another part of the building.

POLLENS. Plants and trees that cause allergy problems have wind-borne pollen that is typically produced in clusters of small, nondescript flowers. By contrast, plants that rely on insects rather than wind for pollination generally have larger,

Animals in the Closet

On rare occasions, a child's allergic symptoms may be traced to animal hair in clothing and furnishings. For example, small amounts of rabbit (angora rabbit), goat (mohair, cashmere), and alpaca fleece are sometimes blended in to soften synthetic yarns. Camel hair is a popular fabric. Horsehair is still used for fine upholstery fabrics and as an interfacing in some tailored garments. Fur trimmings and linings may cause problems; doll hair and toys imported from abroad may contain animal fur or other unlabeled natural materials. Read labels carefully and, when in doubt, don't buy.

bright, showy flowers and are less allergenic. In general, the prettier the plant, the less likely it is to be allergenic. Children with allergies to insect venom should keep away from bright flowers that attract bees (also see Chapter 6, "Killer Allergies: Anaphylaxis").

Pollen counts rise and lead to symptoms when the weather is dry, warm, and breezy. But people with hay fever and asthma may also find that their symptoms worsen during thunderstorms, when atmospheric conditions help to break down pollen grains, releasing allergen-bearing granules. No matter how high or low the pollen count, daily outdoor pollen levels are highest, on average, between midmorning and late afternoon. It's a good idea to concentrate on indoor activities during pollen season, especially if you can keep the windows shut and the air conditioner running.

MOLDS AND FUNGI. Spores from molds and fungi get less attention than pollens, although they may be a very important cause of allergies. When air samples are measured for pollen and spore counts, spores are usually much more numerous than pollen grains. Spores are in the air all year long. Damp, mild weather promotes mold and fungus growth; warm, breezy weather favors circulation of spores on air currents. A mold-allergic youngster has a good excuse for avoiding outdoor chores that stir up molds in decomposing plant material, such as raking lawn clippings and fallen leaves.

While molds are everywhere outdoors, they are also common indoors, especially where the humidity is above 40 percent. Molds thrive on organic materials, such as wood, cotton and other natural fibers, wicker, straw, paper, and leather. Mildew, another name for mold, is almost always a problem in bathrooms. Dried flower arrangements not only gather dust, but also harbor high mold counts. Molds are highly opportunistic and, given the right amount of moisture in the air, can gain a foothold even on man-made surfaces that offer no other source of nutrition.

To discourage molds and fungi, clean household surfaces regularly with an ammonia-based cleaner, diluted household bleach, and/or an antibacterial spray, and keep indoor humidity below 40 percent. Shy away from using humidifiers. Any area of your home that has been damaged by water can harbor mold; if there are leaks (in the roof, for example), find and seal them.

MEDICATIONS TO SUPPRESS SYMPTOMS

Several effective, easy-to-use medications are available to treat allergy symptoms. Some are available by prescription and others over the counter. As with any medications, over-the-counter products should be used only with the advice of your child's pediatrician.

ANTIHISTAMINES. Antihistamines, the longest-established allergy medications, dampen the allergic reaction mainly by suppressing the effects of histamine (itching, swelling, and mucus production) in the tissues. For mild allergy symptoms, your pediatrician may recommend one of the antihistamines widely available over the counter. Children who don't like to swallow tablets may prefer the medication in syrup form. All the over-the-counter antihistamines have drowsiness as a possible side effect. For this reason, it's best to give the dose in the evening, which can both relieve symptoms and help your child with allergies sleep better. However, there are now newer antihistamines that do not cause drowsiness.

Available only by prescription, they are especially useful for school-age children, who need to remain alert during the daytime. Ask your pediatrician whether these nonsedating antihistamines are appropriate for your child.

Antihistamines can be useful for controlling the itchiness that accompanies hay fever, eczema, and hives. Your pediatrician may advise your child to take them regularly or just as needed. However, antihistamines work best when taken every day rather than intermittently. The newer prescription antihistamines have the convenience of once-a-day dosing, which makes it easy for children to use them daily. A new antihistamine nasal spray is available for hay fever. It works in the nose to reduce symptoms, but it has to be used two or three times a day.

DECONGESTANTS. For hay fever sufferers, antihistamines help stop runny nose, itching, and sneezing, but they have little effect on stuffiness. To cover the range of symptoms, an antihistamine is often given together with a decongestant, sometimes combined in a single medication. In contrast to the older antihistamines, which tend to make people sleepy, decongestants taken by mouth can cause stimulation. Children taking these medications may act "hyper," feel anxious, have a racing heart, or find it difficult to get to sleep.

Decongestant treatment can be given topically with nose drops or sprays, but these medications have to be used carefully, because prolonged use can lead to a rebound effect. The resulting stuffy nose is more difficult to treat than the original allergy symptoms.

Cromolyn sodium, best known as an anti-asthma medication (see table, p. 136), is sometimes recommended to prevent nasal allergy symptoms. This medication can be used either every day for chronic problems or just for a limited period when a child is likely to encounter allergens. The medication is available without prescription as a spray; it is taken three or four times a day.

CORTICOSTEROIDS. Corticosteroids—a category of medications also called "steroids" or "cortisones"—are highly effective for allergy treatment and are widely used to stop symptoms. They are available as creams (ointments), nasal sprays, asthma sprays, and pills or liquids. Steroid creams are a mainstay of treatment for children with eczema. As long as they are used sparingly, at the lowest strength that does the job, steroid creams are very safe and effective. They control the rash when applied twice a day, or even once a day if the rash is not severe. Nasal sprays that contain a compound derived from cortisone have become the most effective form of treatment for patients with nasal allergy problems. Once- or twice-a-day dosing is usually enough. These medications work best if used on a regular daily schedule, rather than with as-needed, interrupted dosing. No problems have emerged in patients using cortisone nasal sprays over the long term. Corticosteroid asthma inhalers are frequently used for treatment of asthma and, like steroid nasal sprays, are effective in controlling symptoms (also see Chapter 11, "Approaches to Asthma Treatments").

Steroid pills or liquid are sometimes used for short periods to bring allergy or asthma symptoms under control so that other measures can have a chance to work. In rare cases, a child may have to take oral steroids every day or on alternate days to control severe allergy problems. Steroid pills and liquid should be used sparingly because they carry a higher risk of side effects, including weight gain, high blood pressure, cataracts, slowing of growth, and others.

ALLERGY IMMUNOTHERAPY. Immunotherapy, or allergy shots, may be recommended to reduce your child's sensitivity to airborne allergens. Not every allergy problem can or needs to be treated with allergy shots, but treatment of respiratory allergies to pollen, dust mites, and outdoor molds is often successful. In special circumstances, immunotherapy for a cat allergy can be attempted (say, for a veterinarian who has to earn a living by treating cats), but allergy specialists strongly advise that avoidance is the best way to manage cat allergy in children.

Immunotherapy takes some time to work and demands patience and commitment. The treatment is given by injecting gradually stronger doses of allergen extract once or twice a week at first, then at longer intervals: for example, once every 2 weeks, then every 3 weeks, and eventually every 4 weeks. The effect of the extract reaches its maximum after 6 to 9 months of injections, at which time monthly injections are given to maintain immunity.

After a number of months, the youngster usually feels that her allergy symptoms are better. Allergy injections are often continued for 2 to 4 years, and then a decision is made whether or not to stop them. Many children do fine after the shots are stopped and have no return of their symptoms.

SURGERY AND ALLERGY TREATMENT

Surgery is not a treatment for allergies, but surgery is sometimes performed to correct a condition that is contributing to severe upper respiratory symptoms. For example, the removal of enlarged, infected adenoid tissue from the upper throat, just behind the nose, can increase the airflow in the nose and eliminate a possible contributing factor in recurrent sinusitis (see p. 40). In some cases, a minor surgical procedure is done to drain pus that is backed up in the sinuses.

Adults sometimes have a crooked (deviated) nasal septum, the wall of cartilage that separates the two nasal cavities. A deviated septum can make it difficult to breathe through the nose. Fortunately, this is very uncommon in children; therefore, surgery to correct a deviation is rarely, if ever, needed.

COMPLEMENTARY ALLERGY THERAPIES

Your child's allergy treatment should start with your pediatrician, who may refer you to a pediatric allergy specialist for additional evaluations and treatments. Some parents also seek relief through complementary therapies. Many such therapies are based on traditional remedies that have not been proven effective by scientific testing. Several complementary approaches (for example, acupuncture, acupressure) have been promoted as alternatives to help alleviate symptoms, but it is unlikely that any could produce natural immunity to allergies, as immunotherapy does. If you are thinking about trying an alternative therapy, be sure to talk to your child's treating physician beforehand, to avoid the risk of interactions between conventional and alternative therapies.

Herbal extracts should never be used unless you first check with your child's doctor, because some may be chemically related to your child's allergens and thus capable of causing or worsening symptoms. A compress soaked in camomile tea may soothe the inflammation and itching of hives, but can produce an allergic reaction in a person sensitive to plants in the aster family. The sticky, clear gel (not the yellow juice) from inside aloe leaves may also soothe the skin. Witch hazel is often promoted to relieve skin troubles; however, it is effective only if it is brewed from dried bark, leaves, and stems, which contain tannins—plant chemicals that tighten and soothe the skin. The steam-distilled witch hazel extracts sold in pharmacies do not contain tannins. Congestion of the nose and sinuses may be eased by breathing steam from water in which cloves, bayberry, or eucalyptus leaves have been boiled. Interestingly, cromolyn (see Chapter 11, "Approaches to Asthma Treatments") is extracted from a plant traditionally used by Mediterranean folk healers to ease breathing problems.

Advice from a registered dietitian may help you to plan meals and find alternative sources for important nutrients when your child is allergic to primary sources (dairy foods or wheat, for example). However, steer clear of self-styled "nutritionists" who use methods such as hair analysis or morning saliva samples to evaluate your child's allergies and general health. Time and again, these "healers" prove to have no scientific training in diet and health. Instead, they often have ties to producers of vitamin and mineral supplements. They are interested in marketing superfluous products, not in promoting health through good nutrition. If your child has allergies related to food, ask your pediatrician to refer you to a qualified dietitian with experience in pediatric allergies.

Part III

Living with Asthma

CHAPTER 8

An Overview of Asthma

Andrew, who just turned 3, sees his pediatrician for his third bout of bronchitis this winter. To Andrew's mother it seems that every time he catches a cold, it "moves into his chest." With each episode he coughs a lot, and this time his mother notices wheezing as well. Their pediatrician confirms the wheezing during the examination. The night before, when Andrew was having difficulty breathing because of the coughing and wheezing, his mother gave him a dose of bronchodilator syrup that had been prescribed for an earlier bout. The medication made a big improvement in the youngster's breathing and helped prevent a middle-of-the-night trip to the emergency department.

One of the surprising facts about asthma is that it is a fairly common disease. More than 17 million Americans have the condition and about one-quarter of them are children younger than 18. The rates are steadily rising, though no one can state exactly why. There are probably many reasons for the increase. Not only are we learning more about what causes asthma, but we also have more accurate methods of diagnosing the disorder and better ways to treat it, even in very young children.

Andrew's mother tells the doctor that after the last bout of bronchitis, Andrew never seemed to get entirely back to normal. He tends to cough when running about, as well as one to two hours after going to bed. Andrew is losing sleep and missing a lot of preschool due to the recurrent respiratory illnesses. This, in turn, means that his mother is missing work because she has to stay home to take care of him.

When the pediatrician brings up the possibility that Andrew might have asthma, his mother is both relieved and concerned: relieved because the diagnosis would help explain his illnesses, but concerned because asthma is a serious condition. Her brother Tim had asthma when he was young, and she remembers how their mother had to stay with Tim when he was in the hospital.

The pediatrician reassures the family that Andrew's asthma is not severe and that asthma easily can be managed with proper treatment. He recommends a regular medication program to control Andrew's airway inflammation.

When Andrew's mother calls her brother to relay the news, she is surprised to learn that although his asthma is much better overall than when he was a child, Tim still develops asthma symptoms when he catches a cold or jogs. It turns out that Andrew and Tim are taking some of the same asthma medications.

At the follow-up visit a few weeks later, Andrew's cough and chest symptoms are much better, thanks to the asthma medication program. He is back to playing outside without coughing and is sleeping through the night.

Asthma may appear at any age; however, between 80 and 90 percent of children with asthma develop symptoms by age 4 or 5. Fortunately, in the vast majority of cases, symptoms are mild to moderate in severity. When the condition is properly managed with medications and environmental measures, most acute, potentially incapacitating flare-ups can be prevented. In the fairly rare cases of severe asthma, there are usually warning signs: The child often has eczema starting in the early months, respiratory symptoms commonly appear before the first birthday, and there is often a family history of asthma.

ASTHMA AMONG MINORITY GROUPS

Asthma is a serious and growing problem among minority groups. About 6 to 7 out of every 100 African-Americans have asthma, compared with a rate of 4 to 5 out of 100 for white Americans. African-Americans also tend to require hospital admission more often and have more severe and potentially fatal asthma attacks. In part, the rate may be higher because African-Americans who have asthma are more likely to live in the inner city, where there are higher concentrations of asthma triggers such as air pollution and dust that contains debris from household pests, cockroaches, and rodents.

Among American children and adolescents age 18 and younger, the rate of asthma increased by more than 70 percent between 1982 and 1994. Overall, the number of Americans with asthma rose by 84 percent during the same period. Although part of the increase may be due to better methods of identifying people with asthma, the rise is real and disturbing.

Researchers are working to find cause-effect links between the increase in asthma and environmental problems. Air pollution may be one contributing factor; more than 60 percent of Americans with asthma live in areas that don't meet federal air quality standards. However, blaming the environment and air pollution is not entirely fair and oversimplifies the problem, since the overall quality of the air we breathe is better today than 30 years ago, when the Clean Air Act was passed.

Smoking is another contributing factor. One American Lung Association study found that children's wheezing attacks could be reduced by 20 percent if parents didn't smoke at home.

Some researchers have suggested that better overall standards of health contribute to the rise in allergies and asthma. As they see it, now that widespread immunization and effective antibiotic treatments have virtually eradicated formerly common diseases—

such as smallpox, poliomyelitis, diphtheria, measles, and mumps—our immune systems focus on other targets. Harmless substances that were once ignored—for example, house dust and pollens—may now be perceived as threats by an immune system that doesn't have enough to do. However, this theory fails to account for the key role played by the immune system in immunization. The immune system forms antibodies to vaccines, thus ensuring protection against repeat exposures to infection.

In the same vein, other investigators note that people today have fewer infections and parasitic diseases, thanks to improved standards of cleanliness and hygiene. These improvements, they propose, cause the immune system to switch from fighting infections to producing allergy antibodies.

A sedentary lifestyle—hours spent in front of the TV or computer rather than in active pastimes—leads to overweight, and youngsters who are overweight have a higher rate of asthma, not to mention an increased risk of diseases in adulthood. Children who spend long periods indoors are also exposed for longer periods to the full range of indoor allergens, including dust mites, cooking fumes, odors, and pet dander. But if they play outside, environmental watchdogs warn, they may be exposed to high air levels of diesel fumes and airborne rubber particles from automobile tires, which are among the many air pollution factors blamed for the rise in allergies and asthma.

Researchers agree that adults and children alike need to identify and avoid substances that trigger their asthma attacks, whether those substances are environmental pollutants or individual allergens. They agree, too, that most fatal asthma attacks occur because the disease is poorly controlled on a day-to-day basis. At highest risk for serious asthma attacks are those who don't seek regular medical care and, instead, resort to emergency departments only after they develop severe breathing difficulties. About 5,000 people die from asthma each year in the United States. Many of these deaths are the result of inadequate general asthma care and occur because treatment is delayed, often because the physician or patient underestimated the severity of the attack.

Despite the worrisome increase in asthma, the outlook for children with asthma has never been better. A number of developments over the last decade or so have led to substantial improvements in asthma care (also see Chapters 11 and 13). We have better tools for diagnosing asthma than ever before. And thanks to a better understanding of the causes of asthma, medications have been developed that are more effective because they are targeted to the specific mechanisms behind the symptoms (see Chapter 11). They also have fewer side effects than older medications. New medication delivery systems are also smaller and simpler to use than earlier inhalers and asthma devices.

As we have developed better ways to diagnose and manage asthma, there has been a dramatic shift in attitudes toward the disease. While nobody should ignore the fact that asthma is a chronic, serious condition, children with asthma are no longer restricted—as many once were—to life as semi-invalids. Except in rare and unusually complicated cases, children are now encouraged to take part in any sport or activity, no matter how demanding, that is appropriate for their age and development.

How the Lungs Work

To understand what's going on in asthma, you have to know how the lungs and airways function in normal conditions. The respiratory system is often pictured as an upside-down, hollowed-out tree. The trunk is the trachea, or windpipe, a wide, fairly stiff tube that links the nose and throat to the lungs. The base of the trachea branches off into two large mainstem bronchi, each of which leads to a lung. Once in the lung, each bronchus splits into several smaller bronchial tubes, and each of these branches into smaller tubes called bronchioles. Each bronchiole, in turn, branches into many pockets filled with thousands of tiny air sacs, called alveoli. Bronchial tubes have a wall ringed with muscle on the outside and an inner lining layer that produces mucus that coats the inside of the tubes.

When we breathe through the nose or mouth, air passes into

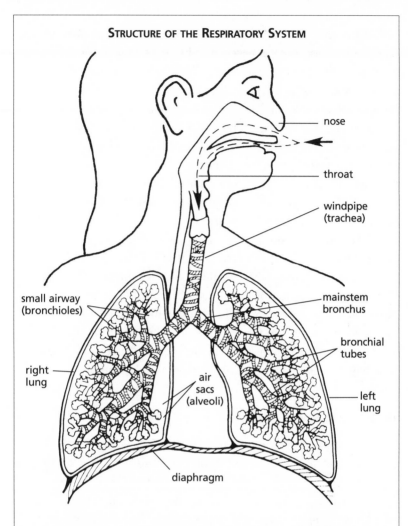

STRUCTURE OF THE RESPIRATORY SYSTEM

nose

throat

windpipe
(trachea)

small airway
(bronchioles)

mainstem
bronchus

bronchial
tubes

right
lung

air
sacs
(alveoli)

left
lung

diaphragm

*Air is inhaled through either the nose or the mouth, and passes through the
larynx (voice box) and into the windpipe, or trachea, a muscular tube. The
trachea branches into a large pipe, the mainstem bronchus, leading into
each lung. Each mainstem bronchus then branches into several bronchial
tubes, which have an outer wall ringed with muscle and a lining that produces a mucus coating. The bronchial tubes split into several smaller tubes,
each of which branches into even smaller tubes called bronchioles. In turn,
the bronchioles branch into pockets filled with thousands of tiny air sacs,
called alveoli.*

the trachea and down through the progressively smaller airways to the alveoli—there are about 300 million of these little air sacs in every pair of lungs—where the actual process of respiration takes place. There, oxygen extracted from the air passes into the bloodstream and then on to all the other tissues. To complete the exchange, waste gases (carbon dioxide) pass out of the blood and back into the alveoli, where they mix with leftover air and are exhaled from the lungs.

WHAT HAPPENS IN ASTHMA?

Asthma throws a wrench into the normally smooth-running airway system. The airways of the typical child with asthma are inflamed, which makes them oversensitive, or "twitchy," poised to shut down whenever they come in contact with an asthma trigger. As a result, the airways in asthma become hyperresponsive. They overreact with constriction and narrowing of the bronchial tubes when confronted with various materials and events to which people who don't have asthma have no reaction. For example, a person who finds himself in a building on fire with high levels of smoke is likely to react with constriction of the airways. This is a normal process believed to protect the lungs. By contrast, a child with asthma doesn't need the extreme conditions of a building on fire to develop airways constriction; he develops asthma symptoms when he finds himself around one of his asthma triggers or catches a respiratory infection.

The tendency to become twitchy is probably present in the lungs from infancy, although in some cases symptoms may not emerge until much later. Researchers generally agree that asthma is a genetic condition; that is, it runs in families and can be inherited in the genes from either parent or from both.

About 70 to 80 percent of children with asthma also have allergies (see Chapter 1), especially to airborne allergens such as pollen, dust mites, animal danders, and molds. Contact with an allergen (for example, cat dander) may set off an acute asthma attack. But when an allergen is inhaled daily at a low level for an extended period (as with mites), this exposure may worsen the underlying airway inflammation so that the presence of another asthma trigger brings on wheezing and breathing difficulties (for more about asthma triggers, see Chapter 9).

New findings have shaken up and overturned many traditional views of asthma. For example, asthma was thought to occur in bouts, with quiet, symptom-free intervals in between. This is only partly true. Recurrent bouts of severe symptoms may be set off by many different asthma triggers, including exercise, cold air, respi-

ASTHMA SYMPTOMS ARE OFTEN WORSE AT NIGHT

Coughing and other symptoms that are usually worse at night are often a tip-off for asthma. However, a fact not generally recognized is that our lungs work less efficiently while we sleep, even if we don't have asthma. Our lung function reaches its 24-hour low point in the early hours of the morning, and this reduction is even greater in people with asthma than in those without.

ratory infections, allergens, or the physical effects of emotional stress. But the accurate picture of asthma is that it is a chronic disease that never completely goes away, even when symptoms are not bothersome.

Asthma is thus both a chronic and an acute disease. First, the airways become persistently inflamed, swollen, and twitchy as a result of repeated exposures to asthma triggers, particularly allergenic ones. The twitchy airways may not be inflamed enough to cause breathing problems, but it doesn't take much to push them into an acute attack. When an asthma trigger comes along, the person with inflamed airways begins to wheeze or, if the reaction is severe, gasp for breath.

In asthma, the passage of air through the bronchial tubes is blocked in three ways and to varying degrees. First, the muscular bands around the airways contract and squeeze the air passages tight. Next, white blood cells enter the tissues and release irritating chemicals that are produced by the immune system (see box, *What Happens During an Allergic Reaction*, p. 4), causing inflammation and swelling in the lining of the airways and narrowing the passages. Finally, the bronchial mucous glands (we all have them, but they are more abundant in children with asthma) overproduce mucus, which further plugs the airways.

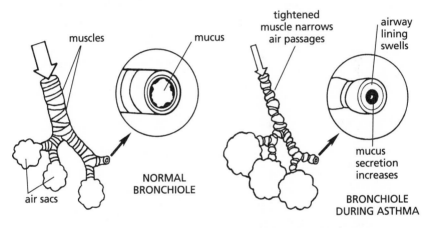

In asthma the muscular bands around the airways contract and squeeze the air passages tight. White blood cells enter the tissues and release irritating chemicals, causing inflammation, leading to swelling of the inner lining and further narrowing of the passages. Finally, mucous glands overproduce mucus, which aggravates the plugging up of the airways.

RECOGNIZING ASTHMA

Many children suffer needlessly because those around them aren't aware of the warning signs of asthma and do not bring the signs to their pediatricians' attention. Asthma can masquerade for years as chronic or recurrent bronchitis, recurrent pneumonia, chronic cough, or respiratory infections. Call your pediatrician for an appointment if your child:

- Wheezes.
- Coughs regularly, especially at night or with exertion.
- Has a tight feeling in the chest.
- Is often short of breath.

Symptoms may not always be there; instead, they may occur occasionally, such as when your child is playing energetically, becomes overexcited or upset, or is sleeping. Perhaps you notice that your youngster wheezes or coughs when visiting a home where someone smokes or has a cat. In that case, keep your child away from that location, and explain to the friend or relative why your child can no longer visit. Never allow smoking in your own home or car. If symptoms come on at particular times, be sure to mention the circumstances to your pediatrician. The more facts he or she has, the easier it is to diagnose asthma and the sooner treatment can start.

MILD, MODERATE, SEVERE: WHAT DO GRADES MEAN?

After confirming the diagnosis of asthma, your pediatrician will grade the condition according to how severe the symptoms are and how often they occur. This information enables him or her to select the right medication and determine the proper dose to keep the condition in check.

MILD INTERMITTENT ASTHMA. A child who wheezes and coughs for less than an hour no more than twice a week is considered to have mild intermittent asthma. Between attacks, a youngster with mild asthma is free of asthma symptoms; nighttime flare-ups occur twice a month at most.

MILD PERSISTENT ASTHMA. In mild persistent asthma, symptoms occur more than twice a week but less than once a day, and flare-ups may affect activity. Nighttime flare-ups occur more often than twice a month, but less than once a week.

MODERATE PERSISTENT ASTHMA. Asthma is classified as "moderate persistent" if symptoms occur daily. Flare-ups occur and usually last several days. Coughing and wheezing may disrupt the youngster's normal activities and make it difficult to sleep. Nighttime

WHAT HAPPENS DURING AN ASTHMA ATTACK?

As an attack happens, your child may begin coughing as she breathes.

Soon she starts to wheeze, beginning with a slight whistling sound and continuing with a shrill rasp as she tries to get air into her lungs. She breathes fast, gasping for air and working so hard that you can see her chest being sucked in on every breath. This effect is particularly noticeable in children, whose chests are small and flexible. The child may appear restless and fearful.

For a child who doesn't yet know how to get symptoms under control and live with asthma, even the thought of an asthma attack is frightening. She panics at the thought of feeling starved for air and struggling to breathe—an action the rest of us can perform without thinking about it.

flare-ups may occur more than once a week. In moderate persistent asthma, lung function is roughly between 60 and 80 percent of normal, without treatment.

SEVERE PERSISTENT ASTHMA. With severe persistent asthma, symptoms are always present, curtailing the child's activities and often disrupting sleep. The child may occasionally have to stay in the hospital for several days to bring symptoms under control. Lung function is less than 60 percent of the normal level without treatment. Severe is the least common of the asthma levels.

MANAGING ASTHMA

How you accept your child's diagnosis of asthma may depend on whether you view life as a glass that's half empty or one that is half full. For parents in the latter category, the knowledge comes as a relief. Finally, they can take the necessary steps to help their child live with asthma and lead a normal, active life. With avoidance of allergens and regular use of medications to calm airway inflammation, most severe attacks can be prevented. Additional medications can be held in reserve to cut off occasional flare-ups. (See Chapter 11, "Approaches to Asthma Treatments.")

Recognizing that asthma occurs in two phases, doctors have changed the way they treat the condition. Now, instead of waiting until an attack occurs, their approach is to control the chronic, underlying inflammation with the aim of preventing acute flare-ups and severe breathing difficulties.

Daily control is the key. Almost every youngster with asthma can be taught to keep symptoms under control, recognize warning signs, and head off serious attacks. Effective medications can quickly stop breathing difficulties. Handy inhalers and nebulizer devices make it easy to take medications to prevent wheezing with measured doses that go directly to the lungs, thereby reducing the risk of side effects (also see Chapter 11).

Severe, potentially fatal attacks occur most often in those whose asthma is not regularly monitored and controlled. Even though effective, convenient treatment is available, too many people still wait until their child's breathing becomes labored, then depend on a visit to a hospital emergency department to solve the problem. Unfortunately, by the time breathing difficulties have set in, it may be too late to stop a bad bout.

Most people with asthma have allergies, and many acute asthma attacks are set off by allergic reactions. Allergy skin tests or a RAST (see Chapter 2, "Establishing the Diagnosis") can sometimes be important in your child's diagnostic evaluation for asthma. Once you know what substances she is allergic to, you can make special efforts to avoid them and thus help prevent many acute episodes.

Asthma Fables and Facts

Although our knowledge of asthma is expanding year by year, many people still cling to outdated beliefs about the disease. Following are some that are often repeated.

Asthma Fable	Asthma Fact
✗ Asthma comes and goes.	✓ Asthma is an inflammatory condition that is always in the airways, even when the person is not having trouble breathing. Exposure to an asthma trigger can worsen symptoms, but the underlying condition never goes away, although it can be controlled with medications.
✗ Asthma is an emotional disorder; it's "all in the mind."	✓ Asthma is a lung disease; it affects the airways, not the brain. It's true that symptoms may get worse when a person is under emotional stress, but this is probably more marked in adults and less so in children. This happens because stress can cause physical changes, including the release of chemicals and cells that irritate the airways. Thus, stress can trigger asthma flare-ups and worsen symptoms. But the effects take place through physiological mechanisms, not emotional ones.
✗ People with asthma should use medications only when they have attacks; otherwise, the medications lose their effect.	✓ Regular use of medications is the only way to calm the underlying airway inflammation and prevent asthma flare-ups. Used at the correct dosage, medications do not lose their effect or cause uncomfortable side effects. Effective anti-asthma medications include inhaled beta-agonists or cromolyn sodium to stop acute attacks and inhaled steroids to prevent most attacks from occurring at all.

Asthma Fable	Asthma Fact
✗ Asthma is just an annoying condition, not a real disease.	✓ Not only does asthma kill approximately 5,000 Americans every year, but the number of annual deaths is rising, despite improvements in treatment. Asthma kills when people do not get treatment to control the underlying condition and stop severe attacks. If everybody who needed them used the proper medications to control symptoms and prevent flare-ups, hospitalizations and deaths due to asthma would be greatly reduced.
✗ Children grow out of asthma.	✓ Most people who have asthma are born with a predisposition to the condition and keep it for life. Many children get much better with age, and their asthma appears to go away completely, only to return in adulthood. Other children never lose their asthma symptoms and continue to have problems all their lives. Asthma should be considered a lifelong condition and requires lifelong attention.
✗ Asthma clears up when you move to a warm, dry climate.	✓ Moving to a place where the climate is warm and dry won't help if a person has problems with allergens that are found there, such as certain pollens and molds. If the proper environmental measures are taken and medications are regularly used, people with asthma can live comfortably in any climate they prefer.

CHAPTER 9

Common Asthma Triggers and How to Identify Them

S ix-year-old Beth has just been diagnosed as having asthma and allergic rhinitis, and her pediatrician has put her on a regular medication program. Beth's parents wonder if her symptoms are related to the house they moved into a year before, her new school, the soccer fields where she often plays, or the cat they acquired after the family moved. Beth has had more problems with her asthma since starting soccer, but her mother can't tell whether the cause is the grass or the exercise. Although Beth never develops obvious asthma when around the cat, her mother notices that the child's eyes itch and her nose is more runny in the mornings after the cat has slept in Beth's room. The house they had moved to is about 40 years old and has wall-to-wall carpeting. Beth's new school was built around the same time.

> *A* sthma triggers are substances that start the chain of events leading to chronic irritation and inflammation of the airways, and may eventually lead the inflamed airways into an acute asthma attack. To keep asthma in control, every youngster needs to identify his own personal triggers and learn to avoid them as much as possible.

To clear up confusion, the family's pediatrician refers Beth to a pediatric allergist, who performs allergy skin testing. Beth, worried that the testing would hurt, is pleasantly surprised to find it isn't painful at all. The test results show that Beth is allergic to dust mites, cat and dog dander, molds, and grass and tree pollen. The allergist explains that children like Beth, who have both year-round asthma and allergic rhinitis, commonly have multiple allergies.

To help reduce Beth's exposure to allergy triggers, the family is asked to put the cat entirely outdoors and cancel plans to adopt a dog. The allergist advises Beth's parents on measures to control dust mites and molds in their home, with particular attention to minimizing these allergens in their daughter's bedroom. Fortunately, the house is air-conditioned, and the allergist recommends using the air-conditioning in spring and summer when the pollen counts are high. Beth and her parents are relieved because they now know who the "enemy" is and—although they have plenty of work cut out for them—they are ready to take action to improve Beth's breathing problems.

— ❖ —

One minute your child is breathing normally as he plays, exercises, or sleeps. The next, he is wheezing, and in no time at all, he is struggling for breath and on his way to a full-blown asthma attack. By now, of course, you know that asthma doesn't appear out of the blue. First, your child's airways become inflamed and "hyperalert" as a result of sensitization. Then, when an asthma trigger comes along, the state of alert erupts into an airways-system shutdown that can cut off the air supply.

Not everybody with allergies has asthma, but the reverse is generally true, especially in children. Odds are that if your child has asthma, he also has hay fever (allergic rhinitis; see Chapter 4) and the allergens that bring on his hay fever are also the triggers for his asthma. In your child's first year or two, he may have had the itchy, dry rash of eczema, possibly due to food sensitivity. Yet, while 70 to 80 percent of children with asthma are allergic, and allergens can inflame the airways, leading them to constrict, not all asthma triggers are allergens. Many nonallergenic substances can irritate the airway tree and prompt the body to respond by

COMMON TRIGGERS OF ASTHMA

ALLERGIES
- Molds
- Pollen
- Dust mites
- Cockroaches
- Animals (especially cats and dogs)

TOBACCO SMOKE

INFECTIONS
- Viral respiratory infections, including colds
- Sinus infections

OUTDOOR AIR POLLUTION

INDOOR AIR POLLUTION
- Aerosol sprays
- Cooking fumes
- Odors
- Smoke (wood fires, wood-burning stoves)

stepping up mucus production and tightening the bronchi. In this case, the body's reaction bypasses the immune system, which regulates all true allergic reactions (see Chapter 1 "Allergies and Asthma Explained"). Nonallergenic factors that often promote and trigger asthma include air pollution, emotional stress, cold air, exercise, odors, and some viral respiratory infections. With both allergenic and nonallergenic triggers, exposure can lead to chronic inflammation and acute and chronic asthma symptoms.

SYMPTOMS-TRIGGER DIARY. Skin tests and a RAST can identify allergens that trigger your child's asthma. However, there may be other irritants that trigger attacks, even though your child is not allergic to them. To help identify nonallergenic triggers, your pediatrician may ask you to keep a symptoms diary for several weeks. You (and your child, if old enough) will use the diary to record the types of symptoms; when and where they occur (for example, when visiting Grandpa, who smokes cigars, or during a sleepover at the home of a friend who has a cat); weather conditions at the time of the attack (dry and breezy, humid and overcast, thunderstorm); how long symptoms last; what action is taken; and what happens to the symptoms after the action is taken. Information provided by the diary can help your pediatrician to focus on unusual or recurrent factors that should be further investigated.

MOLDS. Molds are all around us, indoors and out. They can flourish visibly or invisibly on almost any surface. Often, they can be seen in the form of mildew—gray-black streaks and patches on the bathroom grout or the refrigerator gaskets. Outdoors, they play a key role in the natural life cycle that breaks down vegetation into soil. Every time your child steps onto grass or soil, he sends a cloud of molds into the air. Mold spores float in the air, as pollen grains do. Most of them resettle on new sites, where they can proliferate to form new colonies, but some also enter the airways, where they can promote asthma in a susceptible person. Mold spore levels in the air are often higher than pollen levels, so they are common and important allergens. See Chapter 12 for suggestions on how to control molds and other asthma triggers.

It's impossible to get rid of outdoor molds, but you can help your child avoid the worst of them. While molds hang about in the air in almost any condition, dry, windy weather is the worst for stirring up and circulating extra high levels of mold spores. Check your local newspaper for mold counts, which are usually reported along with pollen counts. Pollen and mold counts are also reported by local radio and TV stations and on the Internet. Plan indoor activities and diversions for days when levels are high.

POLLENS. Pollens are the microscopic granules that fertilize trees, grasses, weeds, and all plants. Different plants release pollen at different times so the pollen season typically runs from early spring to late fall. The cycle begins with trees in the early spring, continues with grasses from late spring through the summer, and winds up with weed pollens in the fall. In some parts of the country where the climate is mild, pollination occurs year-round.

Pollen counts indicate the number of pollen grains circulating in every cubic meter of air. Counts between 20 and 100 are levels that usually trigger symptoms in people with asthma and allergies; however, at counts below 20, pollens can still be asthma triggers. As with molds, it's impossible to avoid pollens altogether. What's important is to take all possible measures to keep from needlessly exposing your child to these and other allergens (see Chapter 12).

DUST MITES, COCKROACHES. In addition to having a gritty consistency that irritates the mucous membranes of the nose and eyes, household dust may contain many different allergenic substances, including pollens, molds, dried-up insect bodies and feces, pet hair, and dander. Perhaps worst of all, dust contains dust mites and their feces (see p. 76), which are among the most common causes of allergies.

Skin testing and a RAST can show whether a child is allergic to dust mites; at least 25 percent of children with asthma have this sensitivity. These microscopic, spiderlike creatures have made their home with humans for so long that it's all but impossible to eradicate them from our dwellings, at least in temperate and warm climates, where the average humidity suits them. However, you can limit your child's exposure to mites by containment measures—confining mites inside their preferred habitats, such as mattresses and pillows—and taking steps to reduce their numbers in places you can't seal off, such as carpets. In Chapters 7 and 12 you'll find suggestions for managing dust mites.

Like dust mites, cockroaches are a fact of life almost every place in the world, especially in urban settings. Although many times larger than dust mites, they share many of the same habits and preferences. In particular, they seem to like living alongside humans, who provide warmth, places to stay, and a nonstop food supply. For every cockroach that makes it to the bright lights, there are hundreds that hatch, eat, excrete, and continue the life cycle in the dark spaces behind the walls and under the floorboards. And when they die, their bodies crumble into powder that works its way into the household dust and is breathed into the lungs, promoting allergic inflammation and asthma attacks. A study of inner-city children with asthma found that more than one in three were sensitive to cockroach proteins. A reliable method of eradicating urban cockroaches hasn't yet been devised and probably never will be. In the meantime, measures to control roaches are suggested in Chapter 12.

ANIMALS. Contrary to what many people believe, it's not just animal hair that causes asthma and allergies in sensitive youngsters. While hair may be a problem for some, dander—the fine scales of dead skin that animals normally shed—and saliva can often be more potent sources of difficulties. Cats and dogs lick people who pat them, thus passing on loads of allergens. They also groom themselves by licking and nibbling, leaving an allergenic saliva coating on their fur.

Finding out that a beloved pet is a trigger for a child's asthma confronts many families with wrenching decisions. The best course—although neither a simple nor a pleasant one—is to find a new home for the animal. For a child whose asthma is under control with medications and environmental controls, it may be enough to keep the pet permanently outside (also see Chapter 7 "Approaches to Allergy Treatments"). Frequent washing and brushing may help to make an animal less allergenic and keep saliva-coated hair and dander from collecting in the household dust, but it is a burden and not always enough to reduce the allergen load.

Birds and small rodents, such as hamsters and gerbils, are occasional sources of allergens, contributing to the chronic airway inflammation of asthma. If you decide to keep such a pet despite your child's allergies, confine the animal strictly to its cage, clean the cage daily, and keep the cage away from your allergic child's room. A youngster with allergies should not take part in cleaning the cage or caring for the pet. Be sure to let your child's teachers know of your child's animal allergies to avoid difficulties with chicks, rabbits, or small rodents that are school residents, or with animals that other children may bring on classroom visits.

ALLERGIES AND ASTHMA: TWO FOR THE PRICE OF ONE

Because most children with asthma also have hay fever (allergic rhinitis) and both conditions tend to run in families, researchers believe that the genes that cause asthma must be located close to those responsible for hay fever. That would help explain why the two conditions are so often inherited as a "package deal."

TOBACCO SMOKE. Tobacco smoke is an important and unfortunately prevalent trigger of asthma. Tobacco smoke acts as an irritant that can both cause chronic inflammation of the airways and nudge inflamed airways into constriction and mucus overproduction in a full asthma attack.

Secondhand smoke is dangerous to all children and is a special threat to those with asthma. Don't allow smoking in your home or car and avoid taking your child to homes where people smoke. If your child complains that drivers smoke in school buses during between-trip breaks (the smell is a tip-off), report it to your child's school and to the bus company. If someone in your family still smokes and is finding it hard to quit, urge him or her to seek medical help and join a support group.

VIRAL RESPIRATORY INFECTIONS. Viral infections of the respiratory tract are among the most common childhood illnesses and are common triggers of airway inflammation and breathing difficulties. The viruses responsible for colds, influenza, and other respiratory infections irritate and inflame the airways. Viral infections may end up stimulating the release of defensive chemicals (see Chapter 1 "Allergies and Asthma Explained"), promoting further inflammation along with the secretion of excessive amounts of protective mucus. A virus that hangs around for several days, as most colds, coughs, and sniffles do, may eventually trigger the typical wheezing and breathing difficulties of an asthma attack.

Lingering aftereffects of viral infections may also interfere with some asthma treatments. Viruses appear to make the the bronchi and bronchioles less responsive to inhaled beta-agonist medications for a while after the respiratory infection has cleared up.

EMOTIONS. Emotional reactions can be powerful triggers for asthma symptoms, but it's a major error to put asthma in the category of emotional or psychological diseases, to suggest it's "all in the mind," or to tell an asthma sufferer to "just get over it." Asthma is an airways disease. Its symptoms are physical and, like the symptoms of many other conditions, they can be brought on or aggravated by emotional changes.

Emotional stress stimulates the production of many of the same chemicals that cause airway constriction. Thus, a change in mood in a child with already-inflamed airways may lead to worsening of her asthma. There's also a purely mechanical effect of emotional expression. When a youngster with underlying inflammation cries, laughs, or shouts, air flowing faster and harder can further irritate the airway surfaces, triggering bronchoconstriction and mucus secretion.

Emotional stress may be relatively important in one youngster's asthma symptoms, but negligible in another's. If your child needs help getting her asthma and her emotions under control, your pediatrician may refer her to an experienced counselor.

WEATHER. Almost any weather change can affect a youngster with asthma. Warm, dry, breezy conditions blow pollens about and stir up the molds that flourish when it's damp. Rain showers wash more pollens from trees and grasses, and wind gusts circulate them. Cold air can be a potent asthma trigger. Atmospheric changes during thunderstorms cause pollen grains to burst and release allergenic particles. When conditions remain unusually still for an extended period, air levels of pollutants can rise to troublesome levels for youngsters with asthma.

As long as your child uses her medications as needed to control underlying airway inflammation, she will be able to take weather changes in stride, and fend off acute symptoms with additional medications as prescribed by her pediatrician or asthma and allergy specialist (see Chapter 11).

OUTDOOR AIR POLLUTION. Air quality is steadily improving, thanks to government and private initiatives to encourage responsible attitudes toward the environment. However, some degree of air pollution is always going to be the trade-off for the thousands of products and services we depend on.

Chemical gases (ozone, sulfur dioxide, nitrogen oxides) and particles in the air not only irritate the airways and sometimes trigger asthma symptoms, but can also make the airways of a child with asthma more sensitive to his other asthma triggers. People with asthma have increased levels of IgE antibodies (see p. 4) in their lungs after being exposed to diesel fumes and smog, which suggests that pollution may increase a person's reactions to allergens such as pollen and mold. Weather bulletins now routinely include air pollution and ozone advisories. If necessary, keep your child indoors as much as you can when there are smog and ozone alerts (see Chapter 12 "How Environmental and Lifestyle Factors Affect Asthma").

EXERCISE. Exercise ranks high, along with allergies, as an asthma trigger. About 80 percent of people with asthma develop wheezing, coughing, and a tight feeling in the chest when they exercise. The underlying mechanism is not entirely understood. One theory has it that during exercise, a youngster breathes harder and faster, sending a large volume of colder air through the airways and drying out the mucous membranes. If the underlying inflammation is not under control, the sudden change can trigger wheezing and coughing. Some children can have symptoms when exercising even when their airways are not very inflamed. Exercise-induced asthma usually begins within minutes after a youngster stops exercising and gradually resolves in 30 to 60 minutes, although in some children, asthma symptoms may start a few minutes into exercise.

This doesn't mean that your child with asthma should not take part in sports and strenuous play. On the contrary, youngsters who exercise regularly and control their underlying airway inflammation with medications generally breathe easier and have better health overall. Sports give children with asthma a good way to develop strength and independence. Encourage your child with asthma to take part in any exercise or sport he likes. Some activities may be better tolerated than others. Endurance sports that demand sustained effort without a break may pose a problem for a youngster with asthma. Outdoor sports played on dusty fields may be extra difficult. However, children with asthma can enjoy swimming, as well as many sports that involve shorter bursts of effort, such as baseball, tennis, and cycling. Athletes with asthma perform at the top level in many sports, including track and field, swimming, basketball, and baseball.

INDOOR AIR POLLUTION. As homes are made more energy-efficient and better insulated, they can also turn into traps for irritants and allergens that make life uncomfortable for children with asthma. In a "tight" house with double-paned windows and high-grade insulation, air does not flow freely between the indoors and outdoors. Limiting outside air may be an advantage for a child allergic to pollens, but the reduced air circulation can be harmful for a child who is sensitive to fumes from cooking or from a gas or oil furnace, perfumes and air fresheners, aerosol sprays, dust mites, pet dander, and the other 101 allergens found throughout the home. A solution might be to use air conditioners year-round to filter outside allergens (also see p. 75). High-efficiency particulate air (HEPA) cleaners can help to clean the air inside the house if they are used in rooms with windows and doors shut. An exhaust hood over the stove can whisk cooking odors and fumes outdoors. Families with asthma may find that life is more comfortable if they eliminate sources of indoor pollution such as wood fires, wood-burning stoves, heavily perfumed soaps and laundry products, and gas ranges (see box, *An Irritant Hidden in Plain Sight: Nitrogen Dioxide,* p. 113). Many aerosol products are available in alternative formulations that are acceptable in allergic households. See Chapter 12 for further suggestions about cutting down on indoor pollution to help your child with asthma.

MEDICAL TRIGGERS FOR ASTHMA

Several medical conditions can trigger or worsen asthma symptoms. Treatment of a contributing condition sometimes improves the respiratory problem.

GASTROESOPHAGEAL REFLUX. Occasionally, a child's asthma may be worsened by reflux, a backflow problem in the digestive tract. Food normally passes from the mouth through the esophagus, a muscular tube, and into the stomach. A ring of muscle at the base of the esophagus, the lower esophageal sphincter (LES), normally relaxes to let food pass and then tightens again to ensure that the food stays in the stomach where it is broken down by acids.

Sometimes, the LES opens at the wrong time and lets the acidic stomach contents flow back into the esophagus, where they scald the delicate membranes lining the esophagus and possibly the airways and voice box as well. This condition is known as gastroesophageal reflux disease (GERD). It is not the same as the normal, painfree spitting up of infancy. GERD is frequently a problem in children with developmental disorders, such as Down syndrome, but can occur in any child. A child with GERD may

AN IRRITANT HIDDEN IN PLAIN SIGHT: NITROGEN DIOXIDE

About half of all homes in the United States have gas-fueled cooking appliances, including ranges and barbecue grills. When gas is burned it gives off nitrogen dioxide, a colorless, odorless gas that can interfere with lung function and cause coughing and wheezing. Nitrogen dioxide is released by a pilot light even at times when a gas appliance is not in use. It is also given off by kerosene stoves and heaters.

If you cook with gas, keep your kitchen well ventilated at all times. Budget permitting, install an exhaust fan over the stove with ventilation to the outside. Open the kitchen windows and close the kitchen door to keep fumes out of the rest of the house.

complain of a sour taste and a burning sensation in the throat; some, however, have no complaints suggesting reflex. Your pediatrician will examine your child to determine whether GERD is a factor in her asthma. If so, treatment of the digestive problem may also improve the respiratory symptoms.

SINUSITIS. Children with chronic or frequent sinusitis (see p. 39) may have asthma that is difficult to control. The exact cause for this is not known. We do know that children with stuffed-up noses due to sinus congestion tend to breathe through their mouths. Thus, the air they inhale does not undergo the normal warming and moisturization in the nose and sinuses. The large volume of colder air may trigger asthma in inflamed airways. Another theory is that the sinuses, when inflamed and infected, communicate directly with the bronchi of the lungs, and this results in constriction of the airways. This communication may take place through the pathways of the autonomic nervous system (the nerves that control the heart muscle, the smooth muscles, including those of the airways, and the glands). Or communication may occur through release by the sinuses of chemical-messenger substances that find their way to the lungs. Treatment of chronic sinusitis may reduce both the underlying inflammation and the number of acute asthma attacks (see Chapter 11, "Approaches to Asthma Treatments").

CHAPTER 10

Asthma in
Infants and Toddlers

Ever since Danielle was hospitalized at 6 months for a bad case of bronchiolitis, she wheezes every time she catches a cold. Now it is winter and 18-month-old Danielle seems to be catching a cold and wheezing almost every month. On their pediatrician's advice, Danielle's mother gives her albuterol syrup, a bronchodilator to open up the airways. The medication helps, but it makes Danielle jittery and "hyper." The doctor prescribes a nebulizer machine so Danielle can breathe albuterol directly into her lungs with fewer side effects. The treatment improves the symptoms, but the episodes of wheezing and coughing are happening more and more often. Twice Danielle needs treatment with oral steroids to get through severe attacks.

> *If airway inflammation in very young children with asthma is not treated, certain youngsters may slowly develop permanent problems with lung function. In addition, untreated severe asthma can interfere with children's growth and overall development.*

The family's pediatrician had initially labeled Danielle's problem as "reactive airway disease." However, after confirming a family history of asthma (Danielle's father had asthma problems as a child) and noting how often problems occur, he changes the diagnosis to asthma. The parents are not afraid of the new label, as they know that good treatments are available. Danielle's pediatrician prescribes cromolyn, a preventive medication to be given with the nebulizer with the aim of preventing the wheezing attacks.

Thanks to this treatment, the attacks now occur less often and the symptoms are less severe. Danielle's mother gives her nebulized cromolyn three times a day, even when the toddler is well. She gives albuterol to Danielle by nebulizer only when it's needed. Danielle does not like her "machine" treatments, but her mother has worked out some fun activities to help Danielle cooperate during the treatment.

A dramatic surge in asthma cases among infants and toddlers accounts for a large part of the recent increase in asthma. For now, we have no satisfactory way to explain the increase in asthma among the very young, although the familiar factors common in older age groups—secondhand cigarette smoke, dust mites, cockroaches, pet dander—may well play a role. Suspect factors linked to the first 2 to 3 years of life include early entry into childcare, an increased rate of exposure to more aggressive viral illnesses, and early discontinuation of breastfeeding. At present, however, there is only one strong indicator that an infant or toddler is likely to develop asthma, and that is a history of asthma and/or allergy in a parent, especially the mother. The trigger most often associated with the actual onset of asthma symptoms is a viral infection, and respiratory syncytial virus (RSV) is most often the virus involved.

Wheezing and coughing are common in infants and toddlers, and doctors are cautious about labeling such symptoms as asthma until they have ruled out other possibilities. In the past, however, reluctance to acknowledge that asthma could affect even the youngest children sometimes led to underdiagnosis of asthma. Instead, infants and toddlers were often said to have chronic bronchitis, wheezy bronchitis, reactive airway disease, recurrent pneumonia, or recurrent upper respiratory infections. Consequently, many children with asthma did not get the treatment they needed. Wheezing and coughing are not always symptoms

Breastfeeding Is Best for All Babies and May Decrease Asthma

The results of several studies have shown that the rates of eczema, food allergy, asthma, and allergic rhinitis up to age 17 are lower in youngsters who were breastfed for 6 months or longer. The beneficial effect of breast-feeding is even greater when families take care to eliminate other environmental allergens, such as pets and household dust.

The American Academy of Pediatrics recommends that mothers breastfeed exclusively for the first 6 months (about the time your baby's diet begins to include solid foods) and continue breastfeeding as long as baby and mother want to do so.

of asthma, but all respiratory symptoms in children should be promptly investigated to determine the cause. Treatment, when needed, should be started as soon as possible.

Why Do Infants and Toddlers Develop Asthma?

Although not every cough or wheeze is a sign that a baby has asthma, recurrent bouts of coughing and wheezing, whether in children or adults, are almost always due to asthma and should be considered as such unless proved to be another condition.

Broadly speaking, there are two types of wheezing in babies under 1 year: nonallergic and allergic. Nonallergic infants wheeze most often when they have an upper respiratory infection. But as these children approach the preschool years, their airways grow larger and the wheezing disappears.

Babies with allergies also wheeze when they catch respiratory viral infections, but unlike the first group, they are likely to develop asthma that will persist throughout childhood and beyond. Allergic babies may have other telling signs and symptoms, such as eczema (see Chapter 3), hay fever (allergic rhinitis, see Chapter

Babies Have Sensitive Airways

All healthy babies are born with highly responsive airways. This characteristic of infants is similar to the airway hyperresponsiveness that is the hallmark of asthma in older children and adults (see Chapter 1 "Allergies and Asthma Explained"). However, hyperresponsiveness in infants is not a symptom of disease, but a normal state that gradually disappears over time unless something interferes with the natural process.

We don't yet know whether or to what extent this early airway responsiveness plays a role in infants' and toddlers' asthma. What we do know is that in normal circumstances, it gradually fades away. In some children, however, exposure to stimuli such as secondhand tobacco smoke or certain viral infections, or a family history of asthma, seems to interfere with the process.

4), or food allergy (see Chapter 5). At this early stage, both groups of wheezers may benefit from asthma treatment. Many in the first group will outgrow the need for medication by about the time they enter kindergarten. Those in the second often continue to require asthma treatment and may need therapy for the other aspects of allergy as well.

Babies and toddlers often develop wheezy bronchitis during the many viral infections that occur during the early years, before the immune system has had time to mature. This tendency generally disappears by the time children are ready for school. The causes of wheezy bronchitis may be different from the causes underlying asthma, and a child can have both conditions at the same time. Of all the babies who have recurrent wheezing in their first year, fewer than a third are still wheezing in later childhood. However, wheezing must always be taken seriously, because almost half of all children with asthma develop symptoms before their first birthday.

As a rule, if your infant has three or more bouts of wheezing, no matter what the cause may be, your pediatrician will consider the possibility of asthma until he or she can definitively rule it out. If tests indicate that your baby has asthma, your doctor will recommend a treatment plan that includes medications, along with an education program. Your pediatrician will work with you to develop a strategy to prevent severe symptoms and flare-ups.

DIAGNOSING ASTHMA IN YOUNG CHILDREN

One of the difficulties of diagnosing asthma in babies and toddlers is that it's not possible to measure lung function in such small children. In addition, their symptoms may not exactly follow the pattern usually seen in older children and adults (see Chapter 8 "An Overview of Asthma"). However, any wheezing or other signs that your young child is having trouble breathing should prompt an investigation. Call your pediatrician if your baby has recurrent bouts of coughing and wheezing, or episodes when he breathes fast and his chest is sucked in on each breath. The airways in babies are so small that it takes only a small amount of swelling or mucus oversecretion to make a drastic change for the worse in the air supply. If your baby has a bluish tinge to his lips or nails, this is a serious sign and he needs immediate medical attention.

Although it's not possible to measure lung function in the very youngest age groups, in most cases, your pediatrician can make a diagnosis after examining your baby, asking you some questions about your baby's medical history and that of your family, and carrying out a trial of asthma medication to see if there is a favorable response.

Your pediatrician will ask whether your baby tends to wheeze, cough, or breathe fast when he has a cold, goes outside in the cold air, is near animals, or is in a place that's dusty or tainted by cigarette smoke. Make sure you tell your pediatrician about any excessive coughing that your child has, even if there is no wheezing, since asthma can be present with coughing being the only symp-

BRONCHIOLITIS

Infants and toddlers sometimes have rapid breathing, a deep cough, and loud wheezing 3 to 5 days after developing the typical runny nose and cough of an upper respiratory infection. Fever is usually present. This pattern of symptoms can indicate bronchiolitis, an infectious inflammatory condition that in some cases is a forerunner of asthma.

If your child's symptoms become more severe or don't start to decrease in the normal 3 to 5 days after she catches a cold or sniffles, consult your pediatrician. In a severe case where the child looks bluish and has difficulty breathing, call the Emergency Medical Service, usually at 911.

After an initial bout of bronchiolitis, about half the children continue to have recurrent episodes of wheezing when they catch colds or other viral upper respiratory infections. In many cases, the wheezing gradually fades away and stops altogether when the child reaches the age of 2 or 3. However, children who do not outgrow the wheezing frequently go on to develop asthma. Your pediatrician will monitor your child's progress and, if necessary, provide a referral to a pediatric asthma specialist.

tom. Your pediatrician will also ask whether you or other family members have asthma, hay fever, and/or eczema, or if there's anyone in the family with recurrent bronchitis or sinus problems.

Your pediatrician will listen carefully to make sure that the sounds your baby is making are coming from the airways of the lungs, and not from the baby's voice box higher up in the throat or from the nose. Sometimes, babies breathe noisily as a result of tracheomalacia, a temporary weakness in the cartilage near the vocal cords. They grow out of this stage as the tissues become firmer. In other cases, babies need treatment for wheezing or noisy breathing as a result of inhaling stomach contents into the lungs after vomiting. If your baby starts wheezing after breathing in a foreign object (such as a bit of food or a small toy) that has become lodged in a bronchial tube, he needs urgent medical attention. Unusual conditions related to airways development or prematurity can also cause wheezing in infants.

Your pediatrician will check to make sure your baby is maintaining a satisfactory rate of growth and development. Most infants with asthma make good progress and are otherwise healthy. If your pediatrician is concerned that your baby may be growing too slowly or failing to thrive, he or she will order tests for conditions other than asthma. Certain tests, including a sweat test to rule out cystic fibrosis (see p. 22), may be necessary when your doctor wants to be sure your baby's wheezing and chest symptoms are not due to a condition with symptoms that mimic asthma.

Chest X rays may be ordered during your baby's first wheezing bout to make sure that there isn't a problem in the lungs. If asthma is diagnosed, chest X rays won't be repeated, as the problem is in the bronchial tubes, which cannot be seen very well in X rays. Your pediatrician is not likely to recommend allergy testing right away for your baby unless you suspect that the wheezing always occurs after your child has been around a certain item, e.g., an animal, or consumed a certain food. However, keep in mind that food allergy is rarely a cause of asthma in infants and toddlers, although it may be an important trigger for eczema (see Chapter 3).

REDUCING EXPOSURE TO ASTHMA TRIGGERS

Babies may develop wheezing when they catch viral respiratory infections—colds and sniffles. In the first year or two, one frequent cause of respiratory illness is a germ known as respiratory syncytial virus, or RSV. Later, rhinoviruses—common cold germs—are the usual suspects. One preventive factor too often overlooked is simple hygiene. Remind family members with colds to dispose of tissues and handkerchiefs properly, and to wash their

Allergies are among the most important triggers for asthma at all ages, including infancy. It seems that for infants whose family history predisposes them to allergies, there may be a critical period—some have described it as a "window of vulnerability"—early in life. During this period, exposure to airborne allergens, such as dust mites, cat dander, molds, and cockroaches, may cause the child to become sensitized rather than to build up tolerance.

It may be possible to delay or block the development of asthma and allergies by finding ways to avoid airborne allergens: For example, use air-conditioning to keep pollens out, take steps to contain dust mites, and eliminate dust catchers from your baby's room (see Chapter 9). Don't bring a pet into the household, or keep the pets you already have permanently outdoors.

And even if these measures don't prevent asthma and allergies, they help to reduce allergen exposure and avoid making your baby's symptoms worse. Studies in adults with asthma have shown that the airways become less sensitive to allergens when strict environmental controls are used to exclude airborne allergens for as short a period as two weeks.

hands frequently with warm water and soap. Ask them to wash their hands before handling your baby.

Some researchers believe that children who have asthma are more vulnerable to respiratory viruses, but this is not known for sure. Because infants and toddlers haven't yet built up immune resistance, they are particularly susceptible to infections, including respiratory viruses that can injure the airway linings and leave them more vulnerable to inflammation. And when young children have viral respiratory infections, their asthma often flares up.

The influenza virus is a powerful asthma trigger, and babies older than 6 months who require daily medication for asthma should be given a flu shot every fall. Unlike other immunizations, flu shots are given yearly because the influenza virus continually changes its structure, or mutates, and new vaccines have to be developed to counter the mutations.

TREATING ASTHMA IN INFANTS AND TODDLERS

In providing a treatment plan for your infant or toddler with asthma, your pediatrician aims for more than simply getting rid of symptoms. A comprehensive treatment plan will encompass the following specific goals:

1. Control symptoms with the fewest medications at the lowest effective doses.
2. Prevent severe asthma episodes.
3. Allow the child to attend childcare, play group, and other socializing activities.
4. Permit normal growth and development.
5. Keep side effects to the lowest possible level.
6. Educate the family and caregivers about asthma and how to manage it.

Treatment for young children, like that for older children and teenagers, comes in three parts: education, environmental controls, and medications.

EDUCATION. Your pediatrician or asthma specialist will provide a written treatment plan, with action plans to be followed at home and at childcare. The education program will explain why your doctor has prescribed the various medications. It will include information that all caregivers and everyone in the family, including brothers and sisters of all ages, can understand.

Give copies of the asthma information materials to caregivers, grandparents, and everyone who shares in the care of your child. Take the time to review the materials with them, to make sure they understand what asthma is and how your child's asthma must be managed. Any time your child's treatment plan is revised, send a copy to childcare and circulate the new written information among extended family members.

ENVIRONMENTAL CONTROLS. In Chapters 9 and 12 there are suggestions for reducing your baby's exposure to the typical allergens and irritants, such as tobacco smoke, fumes and odors, pet dander, dust mites, and cockroaches. Food allergy is unlikely to be the cause of asthma in an infant or toddler; however, food allergy can cause eczema in infancy (see Chapter 3, "Skin Allergies") and is sometimes a forerunner of asthma and allergies later on.

MEDICATIONS. In setting up a treatment plan, your pediatrician aims to gain control over symptoms as quickly as possible, then taper treatment down to the lowest possible dose needed to control symptoms and keep your child comfortable. Medications are given with the twin goals of long-term control of inflammation and quick relief of symptoms (see table, p. 136).

The medications given to infants and toddlers are similar to those for older children; only the doses and delivery systems are different. Anti-inflammatory medications are used to control airway irritability. In the very young, cromolyn sodium is often the first choice and it is given by nebulizer (see *Medication Delivery Systems,* p. 126). If cromolyn sodium doesn't help, your doctor may prescribe an inhaled corticosteroid to be given with a spacer and face mask. Corticosteroids that can be given by nebulizer are under development and will soon be available. Beta$_2$ agonists (for example, albuterol) are given to relieve symptoms. These medications are given by nebulizer, MDI with spacer, or in the form of syrup.

If your baby has mild asthma symptoms less than twice a week, daily medications probably aren't necessary. Your pediatrician may recommend a medication to open up the airways as needed and will advise you what measures to take if your child catches a respiratory virus or another trigger sets off a bout of symptoms. However, an infant or toddler who has symptoms more than twice a week should be treated on a long-term basis with daily medication to control airway inflammation and prevent any long-term scarring of the lungs. Your pediatrician may prescribe another medication as well if acute symptoms should occur.

At all times, your pediatrician will monitor your youngster's

CROUP

A young child who wakes in the middle of the night with a barking, seallike cough and trouble breathing may have croup. Occasionally, croup and asthma can be confused. Usually caused by a mild upper respiratory infection, or sometimes by allergy, croup is an inflammation of the voice box (larynx) and windpipe (trachea). It causes swelling that narrows the airway just below the vocal cords and makes breathing noisy and difficult. Asthma, by contrast, is a problem with the airways much farther down—in the bronchi.

Boys get croup more often than girls. Children rarely get croup after about age 4.

A croup attack usually eases if the child breathes for 15 to 20 minutes in a warm, steamy bathroom or next to a window opened to let in cool air. Your pediatrician may suggest that you use a cool-mist humidifier in your child's room for the next few nights.

Medical attention may be needed if croup symptoms are unusually severe. Go to the nearest hospital emergency department at once if:

- There's a whistling sound that gets louder with each breath.
- Your child can't speak for lack of breath.
- Your child is struggling to breathe.

progress closely and adjust treatment as appropriate. When your child has done well over an extended period, your pediatrician may recommend a "step-down," reducing the dosage to see if control can be maintained with less medication or a different dosing schedule.

Studies in large numbers of children have shown that the earlier a child starts anti-inflammatory treatment with inhaled corticosteroids, the better his asthma is controlled 5 years after the beginning of treatment. When used correctly, these medications do appear to be safe over long-term use.

MEDICATION DELIVERY SYSTEMS. It's difficult to give medications to infants and toddlers; they're small, their coordination is still developing, and they can't be expected to follow complicated directions. The best way to get medication into the airways is by having a young child inhale it. This is usually done with a nebulizer, an electrical appliance that converts liquid medication into a fine mist. Your pediatrician or asthma specialist may also suggest an inhaler that incorporates a spacer device and face mask.

It's very important to use a nebulizer correctly in order to make sure your child gets the correct dose of medication. The mask must be held in contact with the face. If the mask is held a half inch away from the face, 50 percent of the dose is lost. If the mask is held 1 inch away, 80 percent is lost and the child gets only one-fifth the dose of medicine he needs to control his symptoms. When a child is old enough to use a mouthpiece, it's easier for him to take medication and more of the dose reaches the lungs.

When helping your child take medication with a spacer device, if two doses are needed, the doses should be released and inhaled one at a time. If you put more than one dose in the spacer at a time, much less medication gets into the child's airways.

If your child attends a childcare center, a play group, or a nursery school, make sure that the staff includes a medically trained caregiver who knows how to use your child's medication delivery device. All home caregivers should also know how to use the devices.

CHAPTER 11

Approaches to Asthma Treatments

Tyler has always had a tendency to have "chest colds," but when the 6-year-old ends up in the emergency department with wheezing and difficulty breathing, the emergency physician says that asthma was a likely bet.

A week after the emergency visit, Tyler's pediatrician checks the youngster's peak flow value. It is lower than normal. When the pediatrician learns that Tyler is missing a fair number of school days due to breathing problems and is less active than the other children, he prescribes a long-term control medication. The pediatrician tells Tyler's mother that the boy should take the medication every day with an inhaler and spacer device. It is a type of inhaled steroid with few or no side effects.

New treatments and a deeper understanding of the mechanisms behind asthma now enable pediatricians to help youngsters and adults control the condition. With the right medications, used consistently, those with asthma can keep the underlying inflammation in check, stay active, prevent severe symptoms, and avoid emergency trips to the hospital.

Although asthma is gaining strength among the population as a whole, the battle can be won for those who have access to good medical care.

Is the Treatment Working?

You can be confident that asthma treatment is working when your child or teenager:

- Doesn't miss school days.
- Regularly sleeps through the night.
- Participates normally and fully in sports and play.

If any of these three elements is lacking or not fully addressed, then the youngster's asthma is not properly under control and the treatment needs to be revised.

The pediatrician spends some time in the office making sure Tyler knows how to take the inhaled medication correctly. He also refers Tyler to a pediatric allergy specialist, who conducts skin tests and finds that the boy is allergic to both indoor (dust mite, cat) and outdoor (pollen) allergens.

The allergy specialist suggests ways that Tyler's family can modify his environment to reduce allergy triggers. Measures include dust-mite control in his bedroom and putting the family's cat outdoors. The doctor works out an asthma action plan and shows Tyler how to use a peak flow meter. He likes working the device to check his lung function every morning, as his doctor has asked. It comes in handy two months later when Tyler has chest symptoms, which his mother thinks are not really bad. But when Tyler checks the meter, his peak flow is down to almost 60 percent of his best. Tyler starts extra bronchodilator medications. With treatment he is able to stay away from the hospital and does not miss any school. Twelve months later at a regular checkup, Tyler and his mother have lots to be proud about. By following through with the asthma program, Tyler has not missed a single day in the school year. He enjoys normal play and sports. And he has stayed off the oral steroids he needed several times the previous year.

— ❖ —

The treatment of children's asthma is a three-way partnership. It requires equal participation from the doctor, the child with asthma, and the child's family. While your child is an infant or toddler, you as the parent will be in charge of his treatment. As he grows into the preschool years, however, encourage him to take increasing responsibility. This will start to prepare him for the time when, as a young adult, he will be a partner in a two-way treatment alliance with his doctor.

In setting up a treatment plan for your child, your physician aims for the following specific goals:

1. Treatment should calm the inflamed airways to prevent troublesome chronic symptoms, such as coughing and breathlessness at night or after exercise.
2. By keeping airway inflammation and twitchiness under control, treatment should enable the child to breathe freely and maintain normal lung function.
3. The child should be able to keep up with his friends and schoolmates in sports, play, and other activities.
4. Treatment should prevent periodic worsening of asthma and virtually eliminate the need for emergency department visits or admissions to the hospital.
5. The prescribed medications should be easy to use and provide good symptom control with a low rate of side effects.

When the child and the family fulfill their role in the treatment partnership, the treatment should control asthma as well as, or even better than, they expected at the start of therapy.

ASTHMA CAN CHANGE, SO MUST TREATMENT

Because asthma can change from time to time, the way your child's asthma is managed may need to be adjusted periodically. That's an important reason to keep in frequent touch with your pediatrician and report any change that may suggest the need for fine-tuning.

Proper treatment usually involves:

- Environmental and/or behavioral measures to minimize exposure to asthma triggers.
- Medications to control chronic airway inflammation and relieve acute symptoms.
- Depending on the age of the child and severity of the asthma, the use of a peak flow meter to see how well your child's lungs are functioning from day to day.

A WRITTEN TREATMENT PLAN

Your child's pediatrician or asthma specialist will ask you and your child how often symptoms come on and how severe they are. Then, after performing lung-function tests and determining how severe his asthma is, your doctor will probably prepare a written asthma treatment plan (see pp. 123, 143). A stepwise medication approach keyed to your child's symptoms, daily peak flow meter readings, or both will enable you to adjust the medications to stop symptoms from worsening.

Your physician may start medications at a higher level to get airway inflammation under control, then carefully reduce the dosage and/or the number of medications until treatment arrives at the lowest dose needed to maintain control. With this approach, asthma can be quickly brought under control and medication side effects kept to a manageable level.

PEAK FLOW METER

The peak flow meter often is important in your child's asthma treatment plan. This handheld device measures how fast a person can blow air out of the lungs. The results of peak flow measurements warn when medications need to be used to fend off more severe asthma symptoms. Using a simple range of color zones—green, yellow, and red, like traffic lights—the meter can often show when the air flow is reduced even before the child feels any symptoms. When your child is having asthma problems, a peak

Your child's asthma treatment plan is based on his own "personal best" peak flow reading, because every child is unique. Your child's peak flow may be higher or lower than that of another child the same age even though their sex, height, and weight are identical.

To find your child's personal best, your pediatrician may instruct him to use the peak flow meter at the same time every day for 2 to 3 weeks during a period when he doesn't have any symptoms and asthma is under good control.

To obtain a peak flow measurement, have your child do the following:

1. Stand up.

2. Place the indicator at 0.

3. Take a deep breath.

4. Close his lips around the mouthpiece and keep his tongue clear of the opening.

5. Blow once as hard and fast as he can.

Repeat steps 2 through 5 twice more and write down the highest score.

After your child has established his peak flow, your doctor will ask him to use the meter every day on waking and before taking any medications or, in milder asthma, when he is beginning to have symptoms. If your child is supposed to use the meter every day, he should write down the daily scores to show the doctor at regular visits.

flow reading puts a "number" on how he is doing, much as a thermometer shows how high a fever is. Your pediatrician or asthma specialist will show you how to record your child's baseline peak score (see box, *How to Use a Peak Flow Meter*, above). You may then compare this "personal best" against the best of three scores your child continues to record daily. When you see your child's scores drop, you will know that asthma is affecting his airways. By adjusting his medication at this stage, you may be able to prevent a full-blown asthma attack.

Starting at about age 4 or 5, your child can learn how to use a peak flow meter and understand what the colors mean.

- Green means that the air flow score is at 80 to 100 percent of your child's peak; his medications don't need to be adjusted and he may continue full activity.
- Yellow means "caution," just as it does on the road; the air flow is between 50 and 80 percent of your child's personal best and asthma medications should be started or increased to ward off symptoms.
- Red means "danger"; your child's score is less than 50 percent of his peak flow. Have your child take his rescue medications (usually a bronchodilator to open up the airways and steroid pills or liquid to calm inflammation) if it is part of the asthma action plan worked out between you and your pediatrician or asthma specialist. Call or see your physician as soon as possible if the peak flow reading stays below 50 percent despite the treatment.

The peak flow meter provides a reliable way to measure symptoms objectively, but it's still critical that the child and everyone else in the family understand how symptoms occur. Too often, a child has to be rushed to the emergency department because family members either didn't know the warning signs of asthma or didn't take action as soon as he started wheezing, coughing, or feeling short of breath. The whole family should be able to recognize signs that it's time to use or adjust medications to ward off severe symptoms.

ENVIRONMENTAL CONTROLS

Allergy skin tests and/or a RAST may be done to identify your child's allergic asthma triggers (see Chapter 9). Once the results are known, the next important step is to remove as many allergens

Corticosteroids and Growth

Concerns have been raised that inhaled corticosteroids may slow children's growth when used over a long period, but physicians believe that when treatment is properly conducted, corticosteroids do not have an adverse effect on the final height children attain. By contrast, chronic asthma that is poorly controlled is known to slow the growth rate and delay physical maturation in some children. Your doctor will prescribe corticosteroids at the lowest effective dose and monitor your child's growth rate at regular checkups.

as you can from your home (see Chapters 9 and 12). It's impossible to make the place you live in completely allergen-free, but you can at least reduce their number. Studies have shown that reducing the levels of allergens can make a significant improvement in asthma symptoms after a period as short as 2 weeks.

Medications

Asthma medications are given for both long-term control and quick relief. Long-term control medications are used either to calm airway inflammation or control the symptoms of chronic asthma. They include anti-inflammatory agents, long-acting bronchodilators, and leukotriene modifiers. Quick-relief or rescue medications—short-acting beta$_2$ agonists, systemic corticosteroids, and anticholinergics—are given to stop acute tightening of the airways and airway blockage (see table, p. 136).

Long-Term Control

Corticosteroids. Synthetic versions of hormones produced in the adrenal glands, corticosteroids are the most powerful anti-inflammatory medications now available for treating asthma. They can be inhaled for use in long-term control, taken by mouth as pills, or injected (systemic corticosteroids) to get asthma quickly under control when a child is beginning long-term asthma therapy.

Cromolyn sodium and nedocromil. These are anti-inflammatory medications used in long-term therapy of mild to moderate asthma in children. Now produced synthetically, cromolyn is based on extracts from herbs traditionally used in countries around the Mediterranean for treating breathing troubles. Cromolyn sodium and nedocromil can also be used preventively before exercise or when a youngster knows he isn't going to be able to avoid exposure to allergens.

Beta$_2$ agonists. Medications in the beta$_2$ agonists class work by relaxing the muscles that wrap around the bronchi of the lungs and tend to squeeze down and narrow the airways in those who have asthma. Long-acting beta$_2$ agonists are usually prescribed together with anti-inflammatory medications for long-term control, especially for symptoms that occur at night. A long-acting beta$_2$ agonist can also be used to prevent exercise-induced asthma.

Methylxanthines. Theophylline is one of the methylxanthine group of compounds, which are muscle relaxants and nerve stimulants found in coffee, tea, and chocolate, among many other natural sources. Caffeine is a related substance. Theophylline, usually taken by mouth as a timed-release pill, opens up the airways for an extended period. It can be used either alone or together with inhaled corticosteroids. It can be particularly helpful in preventing nighttime symptoms in mild to moderate asthma. Although once used extensively, theophylline is infrequently prescribed for asthma, mainly because it can cause side effects and because the other asthma medications work as well or better.

Leukotriene modifiers. These compounds alter the effects of leukotrienes, naturally occurring compounds that are involved in airway tightening and other symptoms related to asthma and allergies. Medications in this group have been developed quite recently and their full potential in asthma therapy hasn't yet been defined. The two leukotriene modifiers currently in use, montelukast and zafirlukast, are used as control medications. They have only mild to moderate beneficial effects, but are very safe. They are taken in pill form, and a chewable form is likely to be available soon for young children.

QUICK RELIEF

Beta$_2$ agonists. These also come in a short-acting form that is used for the rapid relief of acute asthma symptoms and to prevent exercise-induced asthma in children.

Anticholinergics. Ipratropium bromide, a rapid-acting bronchodilator, may be used either as an alternative to dilate the airways when inhaled beta$_2$ agonists cannot be used, or given together with an inhaled beta$_2$ agonist in severe asthma.

Systemic corticosteroids. These are given by mouth or injection to reduce inflammation inside the airways and speed recovery when a youngster is having an asthma flare-up.

MEDICATION DELIVERY SYSTEMS. Asthma medications can be either inhaled directly into the lungs or taken systemically, that is, by ingestion or injection. Inhalation has major advantages over other routes of taking medication—the major one being that the medication passes straight into the airways, and, as a result, side effects are reduced or avoided altogether. In addition, bronchodilator medications have a much faster effect when inhaled than when taken by mouth.

Several different types of inhalers are on the market; your pediatrician will suggest the one that is most suitable for your child. There are important differences both in the way they are used and in the amounts of medication they deliver to the airways. Your child should be taught how to use her inhaler, and her technique should be checked regularly to make sure she is getting the right dose of medication (see box, *How to Use an Inhaler*, p. 142).

To guard against the danger of overdosing, most inhaled medications for asthma come in aerosolized metered-dose inhalers. The aerosol in these metered-dose inhalers contain the ozone-depleting chlorofluorocarbons (CFCs), which are currently being

continued on p. 142

Antiasthma Medications

Medication	Why used
Corticosteroids (glucocorticoids) *Inhaled:* ▪ Beclomethasone dipropionate ▪ Budesonide ▪ Flunisolide ▪ Fluticasone propionate ▪ Triamcinolone acetonide	▪ Long-term symptom prevention; control of inflammation. ▪ Reduce need for oral steroid.
Systemic: ▪ Methylprednisolone ▪ Prednisolone ▪ Prednisone	▪ For short-term "burst" to get persistent asthma under control. ▪ Long-term symptom prevention and inflammation control in severe, persistent asthma.
▪ Cromolyn sodium ▪ Nedocromil	▪ Long-term symptom prevention or ▪ Preventive treatment before exercise or known allergen exposure.
Long-acting beta$_2$ agonists *Inhaled:* ▪ Salmeterol *Oral:* ▪ Albuterol sustained release	▪ Long-term symptom prevention, in addition to anti-inflammatory treatment. ▪ Prevention of exercise-induced asthma. ▪ Not for acute or worsening symptoms.

SIDE EFFECTS	COMMENTS
■ Cough, hoarseness, oral thrush (yeast infection).	■ Safe when properly used.
■ Given in high doses for too long, may affect growth and have effects on bones and skin.	■ Side effects are less if medication is given with a spacer (see p.142). ■ Different corticosteroids are not interchangeable and must be used under pediatrician's close supervision.
■ Appetite change, weight gain, mood change; given in high doses for too long, may affect growth, and may cause many other serious side effects.	■ Need to start early, but not too early, in the course of an asthma flare-up. Can help prevent hospitalizations and emergency visits.
■ These medications have virtually no side effects. ■ Some patients dislike taste of nedocromil.	■ Medication may work within 2 weeks but needs to be taken for 4 to 6 weeks to see full benefit. ■ Safety is the major advantage of these medications.
■ Racing heart, tremor, jittery feeling. ■ Treatment effect may slightly weaken in long-term treatment, but still effective medications.	■ Not to be used in place of anti-inflammatory medication. ■ May ensure better symptom control when added to inhaled corticosteroid (instead of increasing steroid dose). ■ Inhaled salmeterol is as long-acting as oral sustained-release albuterol, with fewer side effects.

MEDICATION	WHY USED
Methylxanthine ■ Theophylline	■ Long-term control and prevention of symptoms, especially at night.
Leukotriene modifiers ■ Zafirlukast ■ Montelukast	■ Long-term control and prevention given as a single medication or in combination with others.
Short-acting inhaled beta$_2$ agonists ■ Albuterol ■ Pirbuterol ■ Terbutaline (These are available as metered-dose inhaler, inhaled powder, solution for nebulizer, or liquid and tablets to take by mouth.)	■ Quick relief/rescue for acute symptoms. ■ Preventive use before exercise.
Anticholinergic ■ Ipratropium bromide	■ Relieves acute bronchospasm. ■ May decrease mucus secretion.

New treatments for asthma are always under development. This table includes the range available in January 2000; however, your pediatrician will tell you about new medications and delivery systems as they become available.

SIDE EFFECTS	COMMENTS
▪ Stimulation, jitteriness, sleeplessness, stomach troubles, increased hyperactivity in some children.	▪ Treatment must be carefully monitored to guard against side effects. ▪ Not generally used for worsening of symptoms. ▪ Usually an add-on or second-line medication.
▪ Low rate of side effects.	▪ Food decreases absorption; take 1 hour before or 2 hours after meals (zafirlukast). ▪ Once-a-day dosing by mouth is convenient (montelukast).
▪ Racing heart, tremor, jittery feeling.	▪ Treatment for acute airway constriction. ▪ In general, inhaled medications act faster and with fewer side effects than those given by other routes. ▪ Not for regular daily use. ▪ If use increases (e.g., if need to use for symptoms more often than 2-3 days per week), asthma may not be properly controlled; control medication should be started or increased.
▪ Dry mouth, drying of respiratory secretions.	▪ May be used with a beta$_2$ agonist in severe asthma, or rarely, alone when a beta$_2$ agonist cannot be used (e.g., child cannot tolerate taking a beta$_2$ agonist).

MEDICATION DELIVERY DEVICES

DEVICE ■ MEDICATIONS	WHO CAN USE IT
Metered-dose inhaler (MDI) ■ Beta$_2$ agonists ■ Corticosteroids ■ Cromolyn sodium ■ Nedocromil ■ Anticholinergics	Children over 5 years.
Breath-actuated MDI ■ Beta$_2$ agonists	Children over 5 years.
Dry powder inhaler ■ Beta$_2$ agonists ■ Corticosteroids	■ May be used by some children as young as age 4 or 5. ■ Results are more consistent in children over 6.
Spacer/holding chamber (used together with a metered dose inhaler)	■ Children under 4 with face mask. ■ Any child who needs help using an MDI. ■ Should be used when child is on an MDI corticosteroid.
Nebulizer ■ Beta$_2$ agonists ■ Cromolyn ■ Anticholinergics ■ Corticosteroids	■ Children who cannot use MDI with spacer/holding chamber or spacer and face mask. ■ Children having an asthma attack.

HOW TO USE IT	COMMENTS
Actuate while taking a slow, deep breath for 3-5 seconds; hold breath for 10 seconds.	■ Difficult to coordinate firing of device with slow inhalation. ■ If child uses the device incorrectly, most of the dose ends up in the back of the throat. ■ Rinse mouth to reduce amount absorbed by swallowing.
Use device while inhaling for 3-5 seconds, then hold breath for 10 seconds.	■ Suitable for children who have difficulty coordinating MDI use with breathing. ■ Child may prematurely stop inhaling when device actuates.
Rapid, deep breath (1-2 seconds).	■ The child must breathe in hard and fast. ■ Rinse mouth to reduce amount absorbed by swallowing.
■ Actuate MDI into spacer/chamber device, then immediately inhale slowly (3-5 seconds) or breathe regularly. ■ Actuate only once into spacer/chamber per inhalation. ■ If using face mask, allow 5-6 breaths after each actuation.	■ Easier to use than MDI alone. ■ With face mask, enables small children to use MDI. ■ Can increase dose of medication delivered to lungs. ■ Decreases amount of dose left in back of throat and reduces absorption through swallowing.
■ Slow, regular breathing with occasional deep breaths. ■ Tightly fitting face mask for children who cannot use mouthpiece.	■ Easy to use. ■ Good method for giving cromolyn daily to young children and bronchodilator medications during moderate to severe episodes. ■ Relatively expensive; time-consuming.

How to Use an Inhaler

Your child must use her inhaler correctly to get the right dose of medication. Check that she follows steps 1–7 every time she uses her inhaler.

1. Remove cap, hold inhaler upright, and shake it.

2. Tilt head back a little and slowly breathe out.

3. Place inhaler as shown in A, B, or C. (A or B is best; C is okay for a child who has trouble with A or B. C must be used for breath-activated inhalers.) For a dry powder inhaler, use D: Close mouth tightly around mouthpiece and, contrary to aerosol inhalers, breathe in fast.

 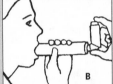

4. Press down on inhaler to release medication and at the same time start to breathe in.

5. Breathe in slowly for 3 to 5 seconds.

6. For A, B, and C, hold breath for 10 seconds to let medication reach into lungs. For D, breathe in quickly; it is not as important to hold breath.

7. Repeat puff according to your doctor's instructions.

Spacers/holding chambers can be useful for people with asthma, especially for young children and those who require inhaled corticosteroids.

phased out. In their place, devices with propellants that do not damage the environment, multidose dry-powder inhalants, and others are appearing on the market (see table, *Medication Delivery Devices*, p. 140).

Tips to Prevent Inhaler Mistakes

- Breathe out *before* pressing inhaler.
- Breathe in through the *mouth*, not the nose.
- Press down on inhaler *at start* of inhalation.
- Breathe in slowly *while pressing down* on inhaler.
- Press inhaler *once* for each breath (one breath/one puff).
- Try to breathe *evenly and deeply*.
- Hold breath for at least 10 seconds. Don't cheat!
- Clean and maintain the device exactly as the manufacturer's written instructions tell you.
- Ask your physician or pharmacist the best way to check how much medication is left.

Asthma at School

In most schools, medications must be kept and administered by the school nurse. This is necessary for children who are too young to manage complicated dosing. It's also important for older children who can't be relied on to take their medications unless reminded or supervised. However, many children are mature enough to keep their own medications and use them responsibly.

When you and your pediatrician or asthma specialist send a written asthma treatment plan to the school, include a written request that your child be allowed to keep his rescue asthma medication in a safe place and use it when he needs to. Whatever the school regulations may require, it's essential that children be able to get their medications as soon as they need them. The worst possible situation for a student developing asthma symptoms is to find that her rescue medication is locked in an administrator's office when the administrator is not around. Children who are mature enough—usually age 8 or 9 and older—should be allowed to carry their rescue inhalers on them (perhaps in a pocket or fanny pack) with a doctor's note. They should also be sure to take their inhalers and medications on field trips.

Physicians treating school-age children with asthma generally prepare a written plan to be sent to each child's school. If your child's pediatrician does not, ask for a written plan that covers:

- A strategy to manage worsening symptoms, including an action plan to make sure the child can quickly get to her medications and, when appropriate, a recommendation that she be allowed to take her own medications as needed.
- An explanation of the medications the child uses for long-term control.
- Measures to prevent exercise-induced asthma.
- Identification of all of the student's known allergens and asthma triggers.

Your child's pediatrician or asthma specialist will probably recommend that daily, long-term medications be taken at home. Any time your child's treatment plan is revised, send a copy, along with a supply of the new medications, to the school nurse.

Your child's doctor will schedule follow-up visits at intervals anywhere between 1 month and 6 months to check on asthma control and determine whether it's time to adjust medications. At every visit, the doctor will ask your child whether there are periods when symptoms are worse and suggest strategies to deal with allergens and other asthma triggers. He or she will also likely check your child's peak flow if the child is old enough, or do a special lung-function test using a spirometer (see p. 20).

ADOLESCENCE

As youngsters enter adolescence, asthma may be one of the many factors that cause conflicting feelings about their emerging independence. At this stage, many find it difficult to accept that asthma is a lifelong condition that requires lifelong—perhaps daily—treatment. They may see an asthma treatment plan as an intrusion on their freedom to choose and act for themselves as they see fit.

To help your teenager build a positive self-image and assume increasing responsibility, your teen's pediatrician may suggest seeing her without the parents being present. In this way, she can be involved directly with her pediatrician or asthma specialist in setting her own treatment goals and working out an acceptable treatment plan. The doctor may invite you to join in and review the plan at the end of the visit, emphasizing your role in supporting your youngster's efforts.

ATHLETES AND ASTHMA

Youngsters with asthma benefit from taking part in sports and physical activity and should be encouraged to do so. However, many experience coughing, wheezing, chest tightness, or unusual fatigue with exercise, caused by loss of heat, water, or both from the lungs when the breathing rate increases and a large volume of cooler, dryer air rushes into the airways.

One of the goals of asthma treatment is to enable youngsters to take part in activities they enjoy without being hampered by asthma symptoms. Of course, your child may benefit from your guidance in making a reasonable choice of activity that doesn't set her up for disappointment or failure because of a high level of associated allergens and asthma triggers. In most cases, exercise-induced asthma can be prevented by taking medication just beforehand. Youngsters who have only minor symptoms with exercise can sometimes prevent them altogether with a lengthy warm-up, instead of taking medications.

Let teachers and coaches know in writing that your child has exercise-induced asthma and may need to use an inhaler before sports. Youngsters who perform competitively at a high level need to talk to their physicians and coaches about medications and prevention strategies in line with the standards set by the United States Olympic Committee.

If symptoms come on while a child is playing at her usual activity level, her long-term preventive treatment may need to be revised. Only in rare cases, where a child has severe asthma or another condition, is it necessary to limit participation in sports. Youngsters who exercise regularly are more fit and better able to deal with asthma than those who are inactive and out of shape.

ALTERNATIVE/COMPLEMENTARY THERAPIES

Alternative healing methods are quite widely used by people with asthma, although there is no scientific evidence that these approaches work. The most popular alternative therapies seem to be acupuncture and acupressure, homeopathy, herbal medicine, and Ayurvedic medicine (an ancient Indian system that includes meditation, herbs, diet, and yoga). Some people continue to consult chiropractors despite evidence from scientific studies that this treatment does not help children or adults with asthma.

Many find complementary healing methods comforting and, in most cases, they may do no harm as long as they are not used in place of the medications and other measures recommended by your child's pediatrician. But potential dangers are that some herbal extracts can interact with medications and a few so-called natural remedies are actually dangerous. Reports in the media and on the Internet can be false or misleading. For example, ephedra, touted as an herbal aid for asthma, hay fever, and weight loss, among many other conditions, is a dangerous substance that has harmful effects and has been involved in numerous deaths. Kola (the same as the cola in soft drinks) can improve airway constriction but, at the doses required, would produce far more side effects than properly regulated medication. Recent media reports claim that high doses of vitamin A can help people with asthma, but excessive doses of vitamin A are extremely toxic, causing liver damage, hair loss and skin problems, blurred vision, and many other damaging effects. Vitamin A supplements should never be given to children except when prescribed by a pediatrician. Avoid herbal remedies and other complementary healing methods unless your child's physician assures you they're safe.

Part IV

Lifestyle, the Environment, and Asthma

CHAPTER 12

How Environmental and Lifestyle Factors Affect Asthma

The idea that asthma is a serious, chronic disease requiring daily management is fairly new. It's not surprising, then, that many families resist the need for daily medication. Instead, they resort to a "crisis management" approach, which asthma experts say is the worst way to treat the condition.

The Gibbons family is a typical case in point. Five of the seven children have asthma. Their mother, Ernestine, stays home and keeps the apartment immaculate; their father, Ralph, is a handyman. The family has no health insurance. Although Ralph works steadily, his wages are low and he earns just over the limit to qualify for the government health plan for low-income families.

Over the years, Ernestine makes so many urgent trips to the county hospital that the emergency doctors and staff know her by name. And while her sick children get

Is there a furry pet in your home? Does a member of the household smoke? And what about all that carpeting?

A big part of asthma control involves identifying environmental and lifestyle asthma triggers and then acting to minimize exposure to them. This means looking for potential culprits in your home. It also means examining your lifestyle for factors that may be adding to the problem.

immediate help for their symptoms, each trip means another bill that the family cannot pay. When the tab reaches $10,000, the hospital garnishees Ralph's wages, which leaves the family with barely enough money to pay for food, let alone buy asthma medications. Each time one of the children is given a prescription, Ernestine divides the dose among any who are wheezing, until the medication runs out and the cycle begins all over again.

Too embarrassed to make yet another appearance at the county hospital, Ernestine turns to the emergency department of a university medical center, where she is introduced to a new kind of asthma care. An asthma counselor enrolls the Gibbons in a free asthma clinic. The children get regular medical care and see the same clinic doctor for periodic checkups. The counselor works with Ernestine and Ralph to reduce many of the asthma triggers that send their children to the hospital. They are put on a medication plan to prevent asthma, and given an asthma action plan to follow. The family also gets help to obtain medications.

On the counselor's advice, Ralph removes the wall-to-wall carpeting, which harbors dust mites. Ernestine stops using air fresheners; she had no idea that their odors could bring on asthma symptoms. The family finds a new home for the cat. They learn to keep the windows shut when pollen counts are high, and apply for a loan to install air-conditioning in the children's bedrooms. Ralph agrees not to smoke in their home or their car. He hasn't stopped altogether, but he no longer smokes around the children and has promised to join a support group to quit smoking.

Although the Gibbons family still doesn't have insurance or permanent medical care, the counselor stays in touch to answer Ernestine's questions and help with advice. Emergency department visits occur much less often than before, and the children's school attendance is better. Ernestine is more confident about leaving home and is looking for a part-time job to pay off the medical bills and help out with the family finances.

— ❖ —

Asthma is the most common chronic disease among American children, and there are many families like the Gibbonses where asthma takes a huge toll. Asthma is the most frequent diagnosis among children admitted to hospitals. It's the reason for more than 2 million visits annually to pediatricians, not counting the other specialists who are involved in asthma care. And while the numbers of asthma cases are rising everywhere and in all segments of the population, by far the largest increase is among people younger than 20 years of age. When all the costs are added up, it's no wonder that this single disease costs the United States $10 billion a year in hospitalizations, doctor visits, medications, and loss of work days.

ASTHMA: NATURE + NURTURE

The numbers of youngsters in the United States estimated to have asthma vary from 4 to almost 10 out of every 100, depending on who's counting. Even at the lower estimate, the numbers are too high. But more telling, perhaps, are the numbers that jump out when the "How many?" of asthma is sorted into "Who?" and "Where?"

GENETIC INFLUENCES. Between 12 and 16 percent of children who live in the inner cities suffer from asthma, compared with 5 to 7 percent of those in suburban communities. Recent surveys indicate that asthma is much more prevalent among African-Americans than among Caucasians. African-Americans are hospitalized for asthma almost three times as often as Caucasians, and their rate of fatal asthma attacks is also almost triple that of Caucasians.

Although Puerto Rican children living in New York City have one of the highest rates of asthma in the United States, similar rates are not seen in all children of Hispanic origin. For example, asthma is much less common among Mexican-American children living in the southwestern states.

In studying genetic patterns among African-Americans, Caucasians, and Hispanics with asthma, researchers have found several asthma-susceptibility genes linked to chromosomal regions that are unique to one or another of the ethnic groups. Much more remains to be done in this area, but the findings to date suggest that genes and environmental influences may play different roles in the various groups. The results may also eventually help to explain why both the number of cases and the severity of asthma differ widely among the various segments of the population. In time, information from gene studies may make it possible to draw up guidelines for better ways to treat asthma in the different population groups.

BOYS VS. GIRLS. Up to age 14, boys with asthma outnumber girls with asthma by a ratio of nearly 2 to 1. There are probably many reasons for the discrepancy, and it may take many years before we find out what they are. However, the size of the airways may be one contributing factor. Young boys, on average, have lower expiratory flow rates than girls, which then switches around as boys grow bigger. They also tend to have more respiratory infections than girls do, and respiratory viral infections are among the main triggers for asthma. Although asthma occurs more frequently in boys, there is no difference in the severity of asthma between boys and girls.

For now, asthma is treated the same way in boys and girls. Perhaps studies on the causes of asthma may eventually suggest that different approaches should be taken.

SECONDHAND SMOKE. Current estimates are that 70 percent of all American children live in homes where at least one adult smokes. Although tobacco use overall is on a decline, a core of smokers clings to the habit, especially in the lower-income groups. Surely it's no coincidence that illness and even deaths from asthma show the greatest increase among children in these groups.

Mothers who smoke are more likely to have babies who wheeze, have breathing difficulties, and need to be hospitalized. Children who come from homes where people smoke make more than twice as many emergency hospital visits as children who are not exposed to smoke. Overall, youngsters whose parents smoke have more frequent severe asthma attacks and need higher doses of asthma medications.

An American Lung Association study found that children's wheezing bouts could be reduced by 20 percent if parents did not smoke in the family home. Don't allow anyone to smoke in your home or car. If someone in your family still smokes, despite everything that's known about the harm the habit causes, urge him or her to get help to quit.

AIR QUALITY. Air pollution has been linked to worsening of asthma symptoms and the rate of hospital admissions for asthma, even though the air we are breathing today is much better than 30 years ago, thanks to government clean-up measures. However, while it's easy to blame air pollution, researchers have a hard time telling where the effects of air pollution end and those of airborne allergens, such as pollen and molds, begin (also see Chapter 9).

The sensible approach is to check the air quality reports in weather forecasts and on the Internet. When the air is bad, follow your pediatrician's recommendations about keeping your child indoors and be extra careful that he takes his asthma control medications.

OVERWEIGHT. The rise in asthma cases is paralleled by a corresponding rise in excess weight among American children. Although there isn't, as yet, a proven cause-effect link between asthma and weight, children who are overweight have a higher rate of asthma than those whose weight is within the healthy range for their height.

Despite widespread efforts to educate families about healthy eating, Americans of all ages are getting heavier. At least 1 American child in 4 is either overweight or at risk. Too much food and too little activity are the obvious causes. Many children spend long hours every day in passive entertainment such as TV/video viewing and computer games. (The American Academy of Pediatrics recommends a daily limit of no more than 1 to 2 hours for watching television and videos or playing computer and video games.)

Provide healthy meals and snacks for your child and encourage her to stay in shape with regular, moderate exercise. If she doesn't like to exercise alone, join her in a daily walk that will be good for both of you. Children with asthma who keep fit seem to have better control of their disease.

INCOME VS. OUTCOME. While many African-American children with asthma live in families with low income, poverty is not strongly linked to the higher number of asthma cases among inner-city children. Instead, there is a direct link between the level of income and the bad outcomes of asthma in these children. One reason is that too many low-income families don't have enough information about the treatments available to their children. Also, too many fall outside the reach of medical coverage. Because they lack regular pediatric care, they tend to rely on hospital emergency departments for their basic health services. To save money and trouble, they may skimp on medications and lose control of the underlying airway inflammation. When symptoms occur, a family may put off taking a child to the emergency department until she is having serious trouble breathing and it's too late for medications to do much good.

Doctors who treat children with asthma warn that this is the worst possible way to deal with the disease. Because the effects of long-term medications aren't always obvious, parents and children alike may think the treatment isn't important. But if preventive medications aren't used consistently, a child is relying heavily on her quick-relief or rescue medications, which sometimes aren't adequate when severe symptoms strike and she can't breathe. Only by managing the underlying inflammation can youngsters with asthma head off trouble and keep the condition under control.

Using a practical, educational approach, many hospitals now provide outreach services to improve asthma care. Trained asthma counselors assist families in eradicating asthma triggers from their homes and adopting preventive measures for long-term asthma control, instead of "putting out fires" with emergency visits.

A priority in most asthma-education programs is helping families with asthma accept the importance of daily control and recognize the early warning signs that treatment needs to be started or stepped up. Such programs have been successful in weaning many families from total dependence on emergency services to self-directed management and long-term control of asthma.

Environmental Measures to Get Rid of Allergy Triggers

Although substandard housing and crowded living conditions are sometimes blamed for the high rate of asthma among inner-city dwellers, asthma is also common among those who live in newly constructed, well-insulated homes and work in up-to-date school or office buildings. Modern construction materials tend to trap allergens and pollutants in a way that drafty little houses on the prairie never did. However, it would be a mistake to try to manage asthma by dropping out of school or living in log cabins.

Some researchers have even speculated that improvements in health and cleanliness may play a part in the increasing incidence of asthma and allergies. According to their theory, the immune system, "bored" because it doesn't have enough germs to fight, tries to keep busy by making enemies of normally harmless substances, such as pollens, molds, and dust mites.

LETTING IN AIR. When it comes to ventilating your home, you may find yourself in a quandary. If you try for maximum air circulation to keep down levels of dust, mites, and molds (see Chapter 7), you may only be opening the doors to pollen-laden air, which can be a major asthma trigger for your child. Asthma and allergy experts recommend the use of central air-conditioning as a compromise, when the family budget allows. An air conditioner is also a form of air filter, which can be useful during the pollen season. With an air conditioner running, pollens are filtered out and the air in your home stays drier, which helps to reduce the mite and mold population.

If you want to open doors and windows to let in outside air, wait until after midmorning, because pollen counts are highest, on average, between 5 and 10 A.M. When pollen counts are high (see Chapter 9), it may be a good idea to limit your child's outdoor activities. After outdoor play, have your child shower and wash her hair. Pollen collects on the skin and hair and, if not washed off, can rub off on the bedclothes and trigger asthma at night.

DUST CONTROL. Among the most common asthma triggers in homes are dust mites, animal dander (see Chapter 7), molds, and cockroaches. Frequent dusting, wet-mopping of hard floors,

Some studies show that air filtration systems help those with asthma; others don't show any significant improvement in symptoms. If you decide to use an air filtration system, you will need to choose between a central and a portable unit. You may find that portable room units have several advantages over central units:

- They usually cost less.
- They can be moved from room to room as your child moves about.
- They can be taken along if the family vacates the home, whereas a central unit may be difficult to remove.
- They can be taken along on vacation or when your youngster is staying away from home.

If you decide on a portable unit, make sure its capacity is large enough to clean the room you intend to use it in. An air filtration unit should carry the following information on its sales tag:

- CFM: The rate of *cubic feet per minute* shows how much air the unit cleans per minute. The larger the CFM rating, the more air cleaned per minute.
- RSP: *Respirable* (breathable) *size particle;* the unit should filter out particles measured at 0.03 micrometers and larger, which is the range likely to settle in the lungs.
- CADR: *Clean air delivery rate* shows the volume of air that moves through, and is cleaned by, the filtration system. A system with a higher CADR number will keep the air cleaner than one with a lower CADR number, no matter what the size the room may be.
- Warranty: Most manufacturers of high-quality units offer a lifetime warranty for central units and replaceable filters for portable units.

and vacuuming sound like commonsense measures for keeping dust and the critters that live in it out of your home. However, dust control isn't as simple as it seems. Several measures to control dust and dust mites in your child's bedroom are described in Chapter 9, and the recommendations apply equally to all the other parts of your home.

Forced-air heating and ventilation ducts can be sources of dust and allergens; in an ideal world, all children with asthma would live in homes fitted with baseboard heating systems or steam radiators, which don't blow warm air and dust through vents. However, since it's not often possible to replace a heating system, the best you can do is take steps to reduce the entry of asthma triggers. For example, you could fit ducts with air filters and clean and change the filters regularly. You could also run a high-efficiency particulate air (HEPA) cleaner in a room with the doors and windows shut. Keep in mind, however, that neither these nor other precautionary measures to reduce asthma triggers have been scientifically proven as effective for everyone with asthma.

Using a vacuum cleaner can sometimes stir up as much dust as it removes (see p. 75). To get real benefit from vacuuming, use only the special allergy bags that are available from vacuum-cleaner dealers and allergy product retailers. The bags are made to fit most types of vacuum cleaners. They are double-walled and have smaller openings to prevent dust from escaping into the air. An alternative is to invest in a vacuum cleaner that is equipped with a HEPA filter.

Vacuuming is not an effective way to get rid of live dust mites, because barbs on their sticky legs allow them to cling to carpets and upholstery. Further, cleaning carpets with ordinary shampoo fails to kill mites and may leave a damp residue that can linger for hours and foster mold and dust-mite growth.

As an alternative, you may try acaricides (mite killers), cleaners, and other products made with either tannic acid or benzyl benzoate, available through allergy product retailers and catalogs (see Appendix 3). Applied regularly to carpets and upholstered furniture, they can help to keep down the dust-mite allergen load.

MOLDS. Try to control molds in your home by making conditions uncomfortable for them. Kill off mold colonies as soon as you find them. Although molds can grow almost anywhere, areas where you're likely to find heavy growths are places where moisture gathers and condenses: bathroom walls and fixtures, shower curtains, under-sink cupboards in bathrooms and kitchens, basement walls and floors, and window frames.

In a family with asthma, it may not be a good idea to bring the outdoors indoors by cultivating plants in pots. Molds that grow in the soil may be among your child's allergy asthma triggers.

Sponge moldy areas with a fungicide cleaner or a mixture of 1 part chlorine bleach and 10 parts water. Throw away rugs and fabrics that have water damage or smell musty. Get rid of carpets and upholstered furniture in the basement and bathrooms, where high humidity generally favors mold growth. To clean a mildewed plastic or vinyl shower curtain, machine wash it along with several towels in hot water with a cup of bleach. Hang it back in the shower to drip dry (vinyl and plastic can't go into the clothes dryer).

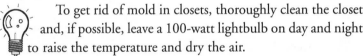 To get rid of mold in closets, thoroughly clean the closet and, if possible, leave a 100-watt lightbulb on day and night to raise the temperature and dry the air.

Keep the indoor humidity level low and avoid using humidifiers. Use a dehumidifier where needed to get rid of dampness. As a bonus, lowering the humidity of your home to below 50 percent, a level that's uncomfortable for molds, will also discourage dust mites. Like molds, mites thrive in warm, moist environments. If you have air-conditioning, keep it running to dry out the air. Clean air conditioner filters regularly to remove accumulated molds and other contaminants.

COCKROACHES. As for cockroaches, if you live in multifamily housing in the city, no matter where you are on the economic scale, it's very difficult to win the battle. Many city dwellers settle, at best, for a truce, or, at worst, for uneasy coexistence. However, in the intervals between professional exterminations, keep

Avoiding Airborne Irritants

Try to keep your home free of the many irritating odors and volatile products that can act as triggers for asthma. Stay alert for irritants that may trigger your child's asthma in friends' or relatives' homes, stores, and public areas.

- Avoid smoke from wood fires and barbecues.
- Watch out for mothballs, room deodorizers, and ammonia-based cleaning products.
- Stay away from perfume departments and shops that carry highly perfumed goods, such as candles or incense.
- Buy unperfumed tissues, toilet paper, laundry detergents, soaps, and other household supplies.

your home clean and free of clutter, such as piles of papers or used shopping bags, that invites the insects to gather and feed. Take care to cover food and wipe up spills.

Aerosol insecticides should not be used in a home where a child with asthma lives. Instead, use sticky traps—"roach motels"—and sprinkle trails of boric acid powder, where you can reach, around water pipes and in other hard-to-get-at places where roaches nest. Boric acid, a mild germicide, is not toxic to humans, but watch that the powder isn't in places where it can irritate your child's airways. Use insecticide bombs only if you can keep your child out of your home while the bomb is active and for several hours afterward, until the rooms have been thoroughly aired and the odor is completely gone.

CHAPTER 13

Teaching Your Child the Basics of Self-Care

Jason's parents remind him many times to take the asthma controller medication his doctor prescribed. But Jason, a typical teenager, just isn't interested. When he feels symptoms coming on, he relies on his rescue inhaler. In time, Jason's parents quit nagging him about the controller medication, since Jason seems to get by. Once in a while, however, he leaves home without checking that his rescue spray is in his pocket. Right away, he begins to feel anxious and his palms get sweaty; obviously, he is heavily dependent on the rescue medication.

A severe attack at Halloween finally convinces Jason that his parents and doctor have been right all along about preventive medications. While he is at a friend's party, he begins to have asthma symptoms that are not relieved by his rescue inhaler.

When your child is young, asthma prevention and treatment are your responsibility. But as a youngster matures, he needs opportunities to assume increasing responsibility for managing his asthma. What he learns, as time goes on, is that he can control his asthma and not be controlled by it.

He continues trying it, hoping the medicine will kick in, but it never does. Jason has heard about people having severe attacks and even dying from their asthma, but he thinks that this is some-

Five Degrees of Asthma Management

The following five steps of asthma management were adapted from a guide developed by Dr. Thomas Plaut, a physician and author who has helped thousands of children and adults control their asthma. The five stages are:

Stage 1—No knowledge
- Cannot recognize an asthma episode.
- Knows nothing about asthma medications.

Stage 2—Beginner
- Can recognize an asthma episode but cannot judge severity.
- Needs help in deciding when to start medication.
- Cannot communicate clearly with doctor or nurse by phone.

Stage 3—Intermediate
- Can handle an episode well with doctor's help.
- Knows how to judge severity of an episode and use a peak flow meter.
- Knows when to start medications.
- Can communicate clearly with doctor or nurse by phone.
- Has made some environmental changes to reduce asthma triggers.

---

thing that happens to other people, not him. As his breathing becomes more labored, it dawns on Jason's friends that the wheezing and gasping are not part of his Halloween disguise. They take him to the emergency department. Jason has to spend four days in the hospital, including 24 hours in the ICU for intensive asthma therapy. After this experience, Jason and his parents are determined to make sure he never has another one like it. Jason begins to take his daily controller medication and to use a peak flow meter to monitor his asthma. It isn't really hard for Jason to stay on his treatment program; all it takes is a few minutes each morning and night.

The whole family has learned how important it is to take a preventive approach by controlling Jason's bronchial inflammation with daily medication. Using the peak flow meter is actually interesting, as well as helpful in letting him know when his asthma control is slipping.

Jason's need for the rapid-relief medication that he used to "live off" drops way down as he follows through with the daily treatment plan. Jason no longer feels nervous if he leaves home without his rescue inhaler. After a while, Jason's parents don't need to check on whether he takes his medication. Jason has grown up a lot; he has become much more responsible for his asthma care and much less dependent on his parents. And whenever the teenager is tempted to skip a treatment, a flashback to his time in the ICU renews his determination to stay out of the hospital.

You, as the parent, are totally responsible for the management of your child's asthma when he is very young. However, in ideal circumstances, your child would progress steadily upward from Stage 1: No knowledge, reaching Stage 5: Expert, by his late teens (see table, *Five Degress of Asthma Management*, p. 160). In reality, of course, the ability to take charge of asthma management is subject to many variables, including each person's emotional maturity. There are plenty of young adolescents who are willing and able to assume responsibility for their own asthma treatment. By contrast, there will always be some rebellious teenagers and emotionally immature adults who may never achieve good control because they refuse to face facts and accept the need for a systematic approach to the disease.

As the parent of a child with asthma, you will progress along with your child, starting with total responsibility for all aspects of care and prevention and gradually handing over more and more of the treatment package. With asthma care, as with other aspects of your child's drive toward independence, you may sometimes find it difficult to give her the freedom she wants. Or your child may progress in stops and starts, alternately demanding more responsibility than she can handle and regressing to clinginess and overdependence for a while.

As noted, during adolescence, asthma management can be complicated by various emotional conflicts—feelings of invincibility, rebelliousness, and risk-taking, among others. While it may sometimes be difficult, keep the lines of communication open, and help the adolescent gain independence and assume responsibility for his or her asthma management. If tensions and conflicts threaten to disrupt your youngster's asthma treatment, ask your pediatrician for some unbiased advice, or perhaps for a referral to an experienced family counselor. Asthma support groups provide opportunities for parents and children with asthma to learn that others share their difficulties. Those who take part may have practical suggestions for heading off trouble or improving a deteriorating situation. Ask your pediatrician to put you in touch with a local support group, or contact a national organization such as the Asthma and Allergy Foundation of America or the American Lung Association, which can suggest resources in your area; see Appendix 2 for national resources.

COMMUNICATION AMONG FAMILY MEMBERS

Although one family member's asthma may affect everyone in the family one way or another, it shouldn't be allowed to limit the family's activities. If a sibling feels she's being neglected for the sake of another with asthma, she's likely to develop a smoldering resentment that may lead to deep emotional rifts.

Clear communication helps family members of every generation—grandparents to toddlers—understand how asthma occurs and why medications and environmental measures are required to keep it under control. Booklets, the child's written treatment plan, and videos are useful educational tools. (See Appendix 3 for information sources.) Family members, when properly informed, become sensitive to the warning signs of asthma and can recognize when the child with asthma needs help. When all the family members understand what's happening and how to manage the situation, they are less likely to fall into one of the two main pitfalls: either panicking when symptoms threaten, or ignoring worsening symptoms until the child with asthma is in trouble and can't breathe.

Staying with the Treatment Program

Most severe asthma attacks can be prevented if those with asthma get the proper diagnosis and then follow their treatment plan. When people with asthma wind up in emergency care, it's easy to put the blame on poverty, lack of information, and problems of access to health services. But this doesn't explain why too many children and adults with asthma keep on having bouts of severe breathing troubles even after effective treatment programs have been prescribed.

Asthma treatment can be complicated. A youngster with asthma has to follow many different instructions. Not only does he have to keep in mind which medications and how much of them to take (see table, p. 136), but he also has to know how to measure his peak expiratory flow (see p. 131), use inhalers and other medication delivery devices (see p. 142), avoid asthma triggers as much as possible (see Chapter 9), and recognize when acute symptoms threaten so he can seek help at once.

None of this is easy. Generally speaking, the fewer medications and the fewer daily doses a youngster has to take, the more likely she is to do so. However, children—particularly adolescents—tend to resist any medical treatment program in the following circumstances, all of which are typical of asthma treatment:

- When treatment must go on for a long time—perhaps even indefinitely.
- When medication is used to prevent the onset of symptoms, rather than to get rid of symptoms already present.
- When symptoms don't always follow right away if a dose of medication is skipped.

This is why some youngsters with asthma have difficulty following a treatment plan. They accept the need for using their asthma medications consistently only after severe symptoms have recurred repeatedly when treatment has been neglected.

Many other factors interfere with the success of asthma treatment. For example, family members may not encourage the child with asthma to follow her treatment plan if the medications are expensive or there is concern about side effects (see table, p. 136).

If the child isn't actually wheezing or having trouble breathing, the family may think that medications aren't needed. Families that tend to seek advice from alternative health practitioners (see p. 146) are sometimes resistant to the idea of using medications, especially preventive medications for long-term asthma control when the child is not having symptoms.

The severity of the illness plays a key role: Surveys have shown that youngsters with moderate asthma are more likely to follow their pediatricians' instructions than those with either mild or severe asthma. In the case of mild asthma, they may think that the condition isn't serious enough to warrant treatment. In the case of severe asthma, perhaps they are trying to deny that the disease is present. Or they may become discouraged and feel that the medications don't help. Whatever the case may be, lack of treatment can lead to symptoms and disability.

CONCERNS ABOUT MEDICATION DEPENDENCE

Some people worry needlessly that their child will become dependent on, or even addicted to, asthma medications if she takes them daily over an extended period. The medications doctors prescribe for asthma are different from the types of drugs that cause addiction. Further, doctors prescribe the lowest dose level and the least frequent schedule of dosing, preferring to give only enough medication to ensure a good treatment effect while keeping side effects to a low level. At times, your child's pediatrician will start treatment at a higher dose level to bring asthma under control, then decrease the medication to a low, maintenance level once your child is comfortable with the treatment program.

With the medications and delivery devices currently available for asthma treatment, you don't have to be concerned about medication dependence or addiction. If your child's pediatrician sees that the youngster tends to overuse a particular medication, it's usually a signal that asthma is not under proper control, and not a sign of addiction. What it means is that the treatment plan needs to be revised.

What Childcare Givers Need to Know

It's not unusual for parents of children with asthma to feel apprehensive about leaving their child in someone else's care. On top of all the unexpected mishaps that can occur even in the best-run homes, parents worry that their child with asthma will have sudden, severe symptoms and the caregiver won't know how to take action in time.

To keep asthma in perspective, head off clinginess, and maintain healthy family relationships, it's important to get used to leaving your child in the care of a reliable caregiver. You can feel confident leaving your child for a break as long as you've prepared the child and equipped the caregiver with everything she needs, including emergency phone numbers. Involve your child in the process; she'll enjoy taking responsibility for educating her caregiver about asthma.

Even if your caregiver claims to know about asthma, get hold of an educational video and watch it with her to make sure she has up-to-date information. Write down the four major signs of asthma—coughing, wheezing, fast breathing, and the chest being sucked in on each breath. Review your written instructions about what to do in case your child has any or all of the symptoms while you're gone. If your child is old enough to use a peak flow meter, demonstrate how to work the device and use it to let the caregiver know when to call for help, if necessary.

In normal circumstances, your child's control medications should be scheduled for the time you're at home. Give the caregiver clearly written information about the quick-relief medications: their names, doses, how each medication is given, what the desired effects are and how soon to expect them, and side effects. Review your child's treatment plan with the caregiver and write down all instructions regarding meals and activities, noting treats that are allowed along with any food or activity that's absolutely forbidden. In leaving the usual emergency phone numbers and the number where you can be reached, provide the number of a trusted friend or neighbor as a backup, and let this person know when you're leaving and when you intend to return.

ASTHMA CARE IN DIVORCED FAMILIES

When a child divides his time between divorced or separated parents, both parents need to stay fully informed about asthma and the medications used in their child's treatment. Each household should have a complete set of the child's asthma medications and the written treatment plan, regularly updated. To keep communication channels open as much as possible, both former partners (along with new partners who share in the responsibility for the child) should try to be present together at their child's visits to the doctor's office.

One parent usually spends more time with the child day to day. This parent may be more attuned to the condition and have more opportunities for learning about asthma. However, this information should be shared for the benefit of the child. If ex-spouses have difficulty communicating with each other, their child's pediatrician can provide straightforward information to both sides and help them keep the youngster's well-being in perspective.

Divorced parents sometimes tend to act out anger and resentment toward the ex-partner, using their child's asthma as a reason or excuse. This is unacceptable, and must be avoided. Differences of opinion may arise between ex-partners over the child's need for medication, the importance of avoiding certain allergy triggers, and activities that are suitable for the child. One parent may accuse the other of being either overprotective or too casual with regard to the amount of attention paid to asthma symptoms and prevention. To avoid hostility, which could cause severe emotional stress to the child, parents must try to deal with any differences of opinion in an open and communicative way. Putting the child or the child's doctor between two warring parents is not fair to the child or the doctor, and often puts the child's health at risk. If you have difficulty discussing your child's asthma care, or any other aspects of his care, ask your pediatrician to refer you to an experienced counselor, who may be able to suggest strategies for working out an acceptable compromise.

Appendixes

APPENDIX 1

Hidden Sources of Food Allergens

Potentially allergenic foods may be used in either natural or processed form for the preparation of commercial foods. Allergic children, when old enough, and their parents must make a point of reading all food labels thoroughly to identify both clear and hidden food allergens. Following are some terms to watch for.

LABELS THAT INDICATE THE PRESENCE OF EGG PROTEIN		
Albumin	Globulin	Ovomucoid
Binder	Lecithin	Ovovitellin
Coagulant	Livetin	Powdered egg
Egg white	Lysozyme	Vitellin
Egg yolk/yellow	Ovalbumin	Whole egg
Emulsifier	Ovomucin	

COMMERCIAL FOODS THAT MAY CONTAIN EGG PROTEIN	
Baked goods (most, except some breads)	Lemon/orange curd
	Malted beverages
Baking mixes	Noodles
Batters	Pancakes
Bouillon (cleared with egg white)	Pasta
	Puddings
Candy	Salad dressings (creamy)
Cereal	
Cold cuts (lunch meats, bologna, meat loaf, meatballs)	Sauces (béarnaise, hollandaise, mayonnaise, tartar)
Custard/cream fillings	Sherbet
Eggnog	Soufflés
French toast	Soups
Ice cream	Waffles

COMMERCIAL FOODS THAT MAY CONTAIN MILK PROTEIN

Baked goods	Imitation sour cream
Batter-coated/fried foods	Instant mashed potatoes
Breads	Instant noodles (cream-style)
Cereals	Lunch meats (nonkosher)
Chocolate	Margarine
Cookies	Puddings
Cream sauces/soups	Sherbet
Gravies/gravy mixes	Soy cheese
Ice cream	Soup mixes
	Vegetarian cheese

LABELS THAT MAY INDICATE THE PRESENCE OF MILK PROTEIN

Artificial butter flavor	Lactose
Butter/butterfat	Milk/derivate/powder/
Buttermilk solids	protein/solids
Caramel color/flavoring	Natural flavoring
Casein/caseinate	Pasteurized milk
Cheese	Rennet casein
Cream	Skim milk powder
Curds	Solids
Dry milk solids	Sour cream/milk solids
Full-cream milk powder	Whey powder/protein/
High-protein flavoring	concentrate
Lactalbumin/phosphate	Yogurt

LABELS THAT MAY INDICATE THE PRESENCE OF SOY PROTEIN

Gum arabic	Soy flour/nuts
Bulking agent	Soy panthenol/protein/
Carob	isolate/concentrate
Emulsifier	Soy sauce
Guar gum	Soybean/oil
Hydrolyzed vegetable	Stabilizer
protein (HVP)	Starch
Lecithin	Textured vegetable protein
Miso	(TVP)
Monosodium glutamate	Thickener
(MSG)	Tofu
Protein/extender	Vegetable broth/gum/starch

NONFOOD CONTACTS WITH SOY

Adhesives	Fabrics
Blankets	Fertilizers
Body creams/lotions	Flooring materials
Dog foods	Lubricants
Enamel paints	Nitroglycerin (medication)
Fabric finishes	Paper

MEMBERS OF THE LEGUME FAMILY (RELATED TO BEANS, PEAS, AND PEANUTS)

Alfalfa/sprouts/honey	Lentils
Acacia gum	Licorice
Beans (including black-eyed peas)	Peas (including green peas, dried peas, commercial pea soups)
Carob (chocolate substitute)	Peanuts
Cassia (substitute in curry powders, cinnamon flavoring)	Soybeans
	Tamarind
	Tragacanth (gum)
Chickpeas (garbanzo beans)	
Fenugreek (flavoring in curry powders, cinnamon substitutes, imitation maple syrup, pancake syrups)	

TERMS THAT MAY INDICATE THE PRESENCE OF WHEAT PROTEIN

All-purpose flour	Modified food starch
Bleached flour	Monosodium glutamate (MSG)
Bulgur (cracked wheat)	
Bran	Protein
Cornstarch	Semolina
Couscous	Spelt
Durum wheat	Unbleached flour
Enriched flour	Vegetable gum/starch
Farina	Wheat bran/flour/germ/gluten/starch
Gluten	
Graham flour	White flour
Hydrolyzed vegetable protein	Whole wheat
Kamut	Whole-wheat flour

COMMERCIAL FOODS THAT MAY CONTAIN PEANUTS OR PEANUT OIL

Baked goods	Ice cream
Baking mixes	Margarine
Batter-coated foods	Infant formula
Candy	Marzipan
Cereals	Mixed nuts
Chili	Nut toppings
Chocolate	Pastry
Cookies	Peanut butter
Egg rolls	Soups
Ethnic foods (Asian, Thai, Indonesian, Indian)	Vegetable fat/oil

Adapted from "Hidden" Allergens in Food, by Harris Steinman, Journal of Allergy and Clinical Immunology, Vol. 98, pp. 241-250, 1996, published by Mosby-Year Book, Inc.

Most near-fatal and fatal allergic reactions to food occur when people are eating away from home. A person who is known to be highly allergic should wear a medical ID bracelet or tag and carry an epinephrine (adrenaline) autoinjector at all times. If a family member is severely allergic, it's probably safest to avoid all commercially processed foods unless you are certain that they are made and packaged by a reliable manufacturer. The Food Allergy Network (see Appendix 2) regularly updates information on its Web site about foods commonly involved in allergies.

Sources for Information About Allergies and Asthma

Allergy and Asthma Network/Mothers of Asthmatics, Inc.
2751 Prosperity Avenue, Suite 150
Fairfax VA 22031
(800) 878-4403   www.aanma.org

American Academy of Allergy, Asthma and Immunology
611 East Wells Street
Milwaukee WI 53202
(800) 822-2762   www.aaaai.org

American Academy of Pediatrics
141 Northwest Point Boulevard
Elk Gove Village IL 60007

                www.aap.org

American Association for Respiratory Care
11030 Ables Lane
Dallas TX 75229
(972) 243-2272   www.aarc.org

American College of Allergy, Asthma and Immunology
85 West Algonquin Road, Suite 550
Arlington Heights IL 60005
(800) 842-7777   www.allergy.mcg.edu

American Lung Association
1740 Broadway
New York NY 10019
(800) LUNG-USA   www.lungusa.org

Asthma and Allergy Foundation of America
1233 20th Street NW, Suite 402
Washington DC 20036
(800) 7-ASTHMA   www.aafa.org

Consortium on Children's Asthma Camps
490 Concordia Avenue
St. Paul MN 55103
(651) 223-9573   www.lungusa.org

Food Allergy Network
10400 Eaton Place, Suite 107
Fairfax VA 22030-2208
(800) 929-4040   www.foodallergy.org

National Asthma Education and Prevention Program
NHLBI Information Center
P.O. Box 30105
Bethesda MD 20824-0105
(301) 592-8573   www.nhlbi.nih.gov

National Eczema Association
1220 SW Morrison Street, Suite 433
Portland OR 97205
(503) 228-4430   www.eczema-assn.org

National Institute of Allergy and Infectious Diseases
31 Center Drive, Room 7A50
MSC 2520
Bethesda MD 20892-2520
(301) 496-5717   www.niaid.nih.gov

National Jewish Medical and Research Center
1400 Jackson Street
Denver CO 80206
(800) 222-LUNG   www.njc.org

Sources of Allergy and Asthma Products

Allergy Asthma Technology, Ltd.
8224 Lehigh Avenue
Morton Grove IL 60053
(800) 621-5545   www.allergyasthmatech.com

Allergy Control Products
96 Danbury Road
P.O. Box 793
Ridgefield CT 06877
(800) 422-DUST   www.allergycontrol.com

Medic Alert Foundation
2323 Colorado Avenue
Turlock CA 95382
(800) 228-6222   www.medicalert.org

National Allergy Supply, Inc.
1620 Satellite Boulevard, Suite D
Duluth GA 30097
(800) 522-1448   www.nationalallergysupply.com

Practical Publications on Allergies and Asthma

A Parent's Guide to Asthma
Nancy Sander and Allan M. Weinstein
Bantam Doubleday Dell Publishing Group, 1994
Call Asthma and Allergy Network/Mothers of Asthmatics
(AAN-MA) (800) 878-4403

*Taming Asthma by Controlling Your Environment: A Guide for
Patients*
Robert A. Wood, M.D.
Asthma and Allergy Foundation of America, Maryland Chapter,
1995
(800) 7-ASTHMA
Suggestions for allergen avoidance and environmental control,
with a product review.

Dr. Tom Plaut's Asthma Guide for People of All Ages
Thomas F. Plaut, M.D., with Teresa B. Jones and
One-Minute Asthma
Thomas F. Plaut, M.D.
4th ed., rev. 1998
Pedipress, Inc., Amherst, MA 1999
(800) 611-6081   info@pedipress.com

Complete Book of Children's Allergies
B. Robert Feldman, M.D., with David Carroll
Times Books, 1985
Comprehensive guide for parents.

A Patient's Practical Guide to Allergies and Asthma
Sheldon Spector, M.D., editor. Written by members of the
California Society of Allergy, Asthma and Immunology.
Can obtain from California Society of Allergy, Asthma and Im-
munology, 5900 Wilshire Boulevard, Los Angeles CA 90036
(323) 937-7859

The Artist's Complete Health and Safety Guide
Monona Rossol
Allworth Press, 1994
(800) 247-6553
Information about safety of arts-and-crafts materials used in
schools.

Creating a Healthy Household
Lynn Marie Bower
The Healthy House Institute, 1995
(812) 332-5073
Guide to using less toxic products and methods for cleaning.

*Athletic Drug Reference '96: Compliance with NCAA and
USOC Rules*
Robert J. Fuentes, Jack M. Rosenberg, Art Davis, eds.
Glaxo Wellcome Inc., 1996
(888) 825-5249   www.glaxowellcome.com
Information for athletes, coaches, and physicians.

*The Civil Rights of Students with Hidden Disabilities Under
Section 504 of the Rehabilitation Act of 1973* (free pamphlet)
U.S. Department of Education Office for Civil Rights
Washington DC 20202-1328
(800) 421-3481

Resources from the
American Academy of Pediatrics

The American Academy of Pediatrics develops and produces a wide variety of public education materials that teach parents and children the importance of preventive and therapeutic medical care. These materials include books, magazines, videos, brochures, and other educational resources. Examples of these materials include:

- Brochures and fact sheets on a myriad of health and parenting issues, including allergies, childcare, divorce and single parenting, growth and development, injury prevention, immunizations, learning disabilities, sleep problems, nutrition and fitness, substance abuse prevention, and the media's influence on young people.
- Videos on immunizations, newborn care, nutrition education, and asthma.
- First aid, child health records, and books for parents.
- The Academy's Web site at www.aap.org, which answers questions about child health and also features information on all aspects of child rearing—from injury prevention to teen dating, fears and phobias to car seat usage. All the information on this site has been reviewed and approved by the American Academy of Pediatrics and represents the collective wisdom of more than 55,000 pediatricians.

For specific information or to keep current on new AAP public education materials, visit our Web site at www.aap.org.

Glossary

acute: sudden; sometimes also used to mean short and relatively severe

adrenaline: see *epinephrine*

adrenergic: medication that acts like epinephrine (adrenaline)

airflow: the rate at which air can be blown out of the lungs

allergen: substance that provokes allergy

allergic rhinitis: allergy symptoms related to the nose, including running, itching, stuffiness, and sneezing, that occur periodically or year-round

allergist: a doctor who specializes in treating allergies

allergy: immune reaction to a normally harmless substance

allergy shots: see *immunotherapy*

alveoli: air sacs at the ends of the smallest airways in the lungs

anaphylaxis: severe, total-body allergic reaction that can be fatal if not treated at once

angioedema: nonitchy swelling that is often but not always triggered by allergy

antibody: protein developed by the body in response to entry of a foreign substance (antigen), conferring immunity

anticholinergic: quick-relief medication that works by blocking the passage of impulses through certain nerve pathways

antigen: any substance capable of inducing an immune response

antihistamine: medication that blocks the effects of histamine, such as itching and swelling

anti-inflammatory: medication that prevents or reduces inflammation

asthma: inflammatory airway disease in which airways are over-responsive to stimuli; symptoms can be stopped or prevented by medical and environmental measures

atopy: allergy

autonomic nervous system: nerves controlling certain functions of the heart muscle, smooth muscles (including those of the airways), skin, gastrointestinal tract, and mucous glands

breath-activated: device that releases medication when triggered by the user's breathing

breathing rate: number of breaths per minute

bronchi, bronchus (sing.): large airways of the lungs

bronchioles: small airways of the lungs

bronchiolitis: inflammation of the small airways (bronchioles), usually caused by a viral infection

bronchitis: inflammation of the larger airways (bronchi) of the lungs

bronchoconstriction: narrowing of the airways due to contraction of the smooth muscles (also called bronchospasm)

bronchodilator: medication to open constricted airways of the lungs

bronchospasm: see bronchoconstriction

cartilage: firm, flexible tissue that supports the large airways and other organs

chemical mediator: naturally occurring chemical (histamine, leukotriene) that plays a role in the body's immune response, which can lead to allergy and asthma symptoms

chronic: persistent or long-term condition (usually lasting 6 weeks or longer)

compliance: taking medication and performing other aspects of therapy exactly as prescribed

controlled release: medication taken in a formulation that allows the release of predictable amounts over time (same as long-acting, slow-release, sustained-release)

controller: medication that decreases or prevents the frequency of asthma episodes, usually but not always by reducing the underlying inflammation of asthma

corticosteroid: synthetic form of an adrenal hormone that is used as a medication to suppress inflammation (also called steroid and cortisone)

cortisone: see *corticosteroid*

cromolyn: controller medication that prevents mast cells in the airway tissues from releasing asthma-causing body chemicals

croup: barking cough caused by inflammation of the trachea and voice box

dander: dead skin scales

decongestant: medication to reduce congestion caused by fluid accumulation in tissues

desensitization: immunotherapy (allergy injections) to decrease or eliminate allergic response to a substance

dust mite: microscopic arachnid, a relative of spiders and ticks, that lives around humans and in house dust, and is a frequent cause of allergies; also called mite

eczema: itchy flat rash, also called atopic dermatitis

eosinophil: white blood cell involved in the immune response, especially the allergic one

epinephrine: a hormone (also called adrenaline) produced by the adrenal glands and released in response to stress and other stimuli; a synthetic form of epinephrine is used as a medication to constrict the blood vessels, stimulate the heart, and widen the airways

episode: a period when asthma symptoms occur, the ability to breathe is affected, and additional medication may be needed; also called bout or flare-up

exercise-induced asthma: a form of asthma that is triggered by physical activity/exertion

exhale: to breathe out

flare-up: see *episode*

flow monitor: part of the holding chamber medication delivery device, which makes a warning sound if the person breathes in too fast

food intolerance: nonallergic adverse reaction to food, which does not involve the immune system

gastroesophageal reflux (GERD): backflow of food mixed with digestive acids from stomach into the esophagus, causing irritation that can lead to bronchoconstriction

GERD: see *gastroesophageal reflux*

hay fever: periodic symptoms, especially of the nose and eyes, caused by pollens and other seasonal stimuli, also called seasonal allergic rhinitis

HEPA filter/cleaner: high-efficiency particulate air filter or cleaner that removes very small particles from the air

histamine: a chemical mediator of allergies and asthma

hives: itchy swellings, usually caused by allergy; also called urticaria

holding chamber: medication delivery device used with a metered dose inhaler to hold the medication mist so it is easier to take, better absorbed, and more effective; also called a spacer or extender

hyperresponsive: immune system or airways that overreact to allergy and/or asthma triggers

hypersensitivity: allergy

IgE: immunoglobulin E, an antibody that is formed by the body in response to entry by a foreign protein, that subsequently recognizes the protein as an allergen and sets off the allergic immune reaction

immunoglobulin E: see *IgE*

immunotherapy: injection of small but increasing doses of a substance to bring about desensitization to that allergen; also called allergy shots or allergy desensitization

inflammation: the body's response to a potentially injurious physical or chemical trigger, with swelling, heat, and redness due to the mobilization of cells, fluids, and chemicals into the injured area

inhalation device: device that delivers medication as the person breathes in

inhaled steroid: synthetic hormone medication taken by breathing in that reduces existing inflammation in the airways and prevents further inflammation from developing; widely prescribed for children with persistent asthma

inhaler: device which transforms medication into a fine mist or aerosol that can be breathed into the airways

intradermal: into or under the skin

irritant: a nonallergenic substance that can cause a reaction in the skin, airways, or other organ or tissues

large airways: air passages wider than 2 mm in diameter

leukocyte: white blood cell (also see *lymphocyte*)

leukotriene: chemical mediator involved in asthma

leukotriene modifier: medication that blocks the production and/or effect of leukotrienes in the airways, thus partly stopping the asthma response

long-acting: similar to controlled-release, slow-release, and sustained-release medications

lung-function test: assessment of the ability to breathe in and out, often done in asthma

lymphocyte: type of white blood cell

mask: device that fits over the nose and mouth to improve delivery and absorption of asthma medications

mast cell: a cell that, when stimulated by an allergy/asthma trigger, releases chemicals that lead to an allergy and/or asthma response

mediator: a naturally occurring chemical through which an allergy or asthma reaction takes place

metered-dose inhaler (MDI): device that delivers a predetermined amount of medication, transforming powder medication into an easily inhaled aerosol

monitor: keep track of

mouthpiece: the part of a medication delivery device that fits in a person's mouth

mucus: thick, protective, cleansing semiliquid produced by glands in the airways, nose, sinuses, and other organs

nebulizer: delivery device that converts liquid medication into a fine mist that can be inhaled

objective sign: event that can be seen and evaluated

onset of effect/action: time lapse between taking medication and feeling or seeing its effects

ozone: a form of oxygen (O_3) that causes irritation in the airways; a component of smog or air pollution

ozone layer: layer of ozone in the upper atmosphere that protects the earth's surface from the harmful effects of ultraviolet sunlight

peak expiratory flow: rate at which air is expelled from the lungs when your child breathes out as fast and hard as he can

peak flow meter: device for measuring peak expiratory flow rate

pediatrician: doctor specializing in the health care of infants, children, adolescents, and young adults

pollen: fine cell grains responsible for fertilization of plants and also responsible for causing allergies

pollutant: impurity that contaminates air or water

prick test: see *skin test*

pulmonary function test: see *lung function test*

quick-relief medication: medication that acts rapidly to open constricted airways

radioallergosorbent blood test (RAST): measurement of immunoglobulin E (IgE) antibody to a specific antigen in the blood

RAST: see *radioallergosorbent blood test*

rescue medicine: quick-relief medicine

respirable particles: microscopic particles (1 to 5 micrometers in diameter) that can be inhaled and may cause irritation in the airways

retraction: "sucking in" of the skin of the chest and/or neck

scratch tests: see *skin tests*

sensitization: process of developing an allergic response to a substance

side effect: undesirable or adverse effect of medication

sign: external physical effects of an illness that can be seen and evaluated by an observer

sinus: one of eight air pockets, or cavities, in the bones of the front of the face

sinusitis: inflammation of the sinuses

skin tests: allergy tests in which drops of allergen extracts are allowed to seep through shallow scratches made in the skin surface

small airways: air passages less than 2 mm in diameter (bronchioles)

spacer: see *holding chamber*

spirometer: device used by a doctor to measure airflow into and out of the lungs

step down: method of asthma treatment that starts with higher medication doses to achieve control quickly, then gradually decreases medications to lowest levels required for symptom control

steroid: synthetic form of a naturally occurring hormone that can be taken by mouth or as an inhaled spray to stop inflammation and control asthma

sustained-release: long-acting medication

symptoms: physical effects of an illness that are "internal" or felt by the person involved (see *sign*)

tidal breathing: normal breathing

toxicity: adverse effects of medication

trachea: the windpipe, a firm tube that extends downward from the larynx and branches into the left and right bronchi

trigger: environmental factor that causes the body to respond with allergy or asthma symptoms

twitchy: description of the airways of people with asthma (e.g., overreactive)

voice box: larynx, part of the upper airways between the throat and the windpipe (trachea) where sound is produced

wheeze: high-pitched whistle heard when air flows in and out through constricted airways

white blood cell: cells that work mainly to defend the body from infectious bacteria and invading allergens

windpipe: see *trachea*

workup: doctor's examination and evaluation

Index

signs of, 26
soaps, 30
triggers of, 29
Eggs, 56. *See also* Food allergies.
Egg substitutes, 56.
Environmental controls in asthma, 123-124

F

Feingold diet, 51
Food allergies, **47-61**
breastfeeding, 50, 54
corn, 59
cow's milk, 54-56
diagnosis of, 49-50
eggs, 56
gluten, 59
informing caregivers of, 53
management of, 50-54
nuts, 57
peanuts, 56-57
reducing risk of, 58
soy, 57-59
symptoms of, 48-49
vs. food intolerance, 48
wheat, 59
Food Allergy Network, 53
Food challenge test, 21
Food diary, 21, 49
Foreign object in nose, 43

G

Gastroesophageal reflux (GERD), 113-114
Gluten intolerance, 59. *See also* Food allergies.

H

Hayfever, 8, 15, **35-46**
allergy shots for, 44
animals, role of, 40-41
bedding, 43
colds, confusion with, 38
ear infections, role of, 39
dust mites, 42-43
family patterns of, 36
management of, 42-46
medications for, 45-46
molds, 42-45
onset of, 36
perennial, 37-38
pollen, 37
pain, 37
seasonality, 36
sinusitis, role of, 39
symptoms of, 38
Heating systems, 80, 156-157
HEPA (high-efficiency particulate air) filters, 45, 75, 77, 112, 156
Histamines, 4-5
Hives, 8, **31-34**
clothing, 34
environment, role of, 34
foods, 34
stress as cause, 34
tests for, 32
treatment of, 34
Houseplants, 79-80
Humidifiers and mold, 79

I

Immune system, 4-5
Immunoglobulin E (IgE), 4-5
Immunotherapy, 85-86. *See also*

Sweat test, 22

T

T-cells. See T-lymphocytes.
T-lymphocytes, 3
Tests, **16-22**
   antibody, 16
   blood, 16, 19
   food challenge, 21
   imaging, 19
   lung function, 20
   pain in, 19
   radioallergosorbent (RAST) 19
   reaction to, 18
   skin, 16-19
   sweat, 22
   X rays, 19-20

Theophylline, 134, 138
Treatment plan for asthma, 123
   written plan, 123, 144

U

Urticaria, 32. *See also* hives.

V

Vacuum cleaners, 74-75
Ventilation, 154

W

Wheat, 59. *See also* Food allergies.

Z

Zafirlukast, 138